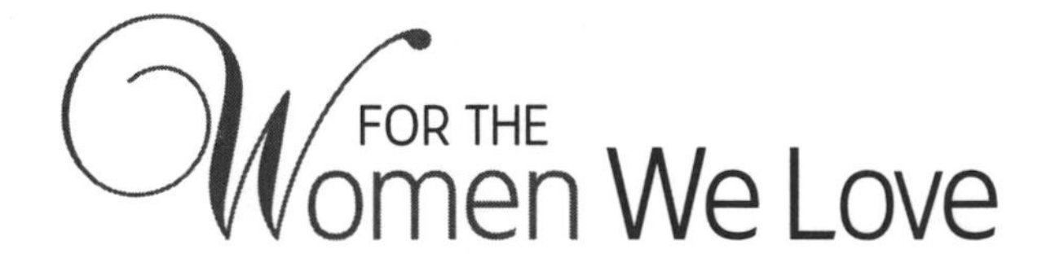
FOR THE
Women We Love

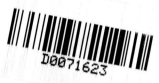

All net proceeds
from the sale of this book
will benefit
Men Against Breast Cancer's
Program Development.

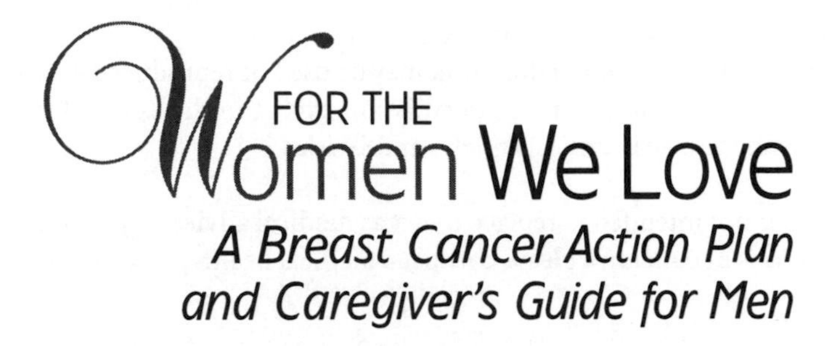

A Breast Cancer Action Plan and Caregiver's Guide for Men

Matthew J. Loscalzo, MSW
with
Marc Heyison,
President, Men Against Breast Cancer

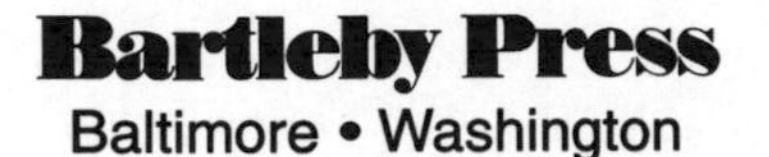

This book is not intended to replace or act as medical advice. If you have any questions or concerns, please contact a medical health professional.

Bartleby Press
9045 Maier Road
Laurel, MD 20723
800-953-9929
www.BartlebythePublisher.com

To learn more about what men can do the fight breast cancer visit
www.MenAgainstBreastCancer.org

ISBN: 978-0-910155-71-7
Library of Congress Control Number: 2007934306

Cover Design by Ross Feldner
Cover Photo by Victoria Prouty
Illustrations by Ralph Butler

Printed in the United States of America

In memory of my sister, Marie, who died from breast cancer but lived a fuller life because of it.

And to my wife, Joanne, who has committed her life to helping women with breast cancer to live full meaningful lives.

—M.L.

To my mom and dad, for teaching me by their own example how to treat people with the respect, compassion, and dignity they deserve.

To my wife, Tanya, and her unwavering and unconditional support in all my efforts. You will always melt my heart.

And to our daughter, Samantha. It brings tears to my eyes when I think how great God is to have given us such a jewel. Words can never do justice to the wonder and joy she showers on us every day. I pray she will always feel safe in my arms.

There really is nothing like family.

—M.H.

Contents

Preface

In March of 1992, I heard these five horrific words: "Your mother has breast cancer." I can't begin to express the fear and hopelessness I felt at that moment. Was my mom going to die?

Today, I am blessed and privileged to do what I do in honor of Mom's survivorship instead of in her memory. Her courage not only kept our family together throughout her illness, but was the fuel that propelled me to become a passionate advocate for others who are navigating the same crisis.

Mom was never alone while she was going through treatment. Supporting her came naturally to our family. Our parents had always taught us the importance of being there for the people we love and never forgetting where we came from. My mom had always been there for us; now it was our turn to give back. She had not raised her hand and asked for breast cancer, so we did not raise our hand and ask to help; we did what we had to do—be there and support her.

As my family and I went with my mom to her doctor appointments, I was amazed to see how many women were there by themselves. We all felt badly that anyone facing a life threatening disease was doing it alone. I could see the fear and apprehension in their eyes, and couldn't understand why they didn't have anyone else's eyes to look into for comfort. Of course, I knew that everyone's situation was different with different responsibilities that could preclude the husband from being there. However, I found it hard to accept that someone else was not there in his place.

Men Against Breast Cancer (MABC) was born in those waiting rooms. I felt strongly that every man should support the woman he loves in her time of need. His commitment should not be optional.

Our goal at MABC is to educate and empower men to be there for women during and after their battle against breast cancer. This Caregiver's Guide for Men provides a blueprint for how to best care for the patient while simultaneously improving the quality of her survivorship.

Martin Luther King said, "Everyone can be great because everyone can serve. It only takes a heart full of grace [and] a soul generated by love." There can be no greater embodiment of this than standing by a family member or friend in need.

As I became more active in my breast cancer advocacy, I began to travel the country to meet people who were struggling with this horrible disease, both on the health care side and patient side. I learned many things on these visits, but most of all that the real heroes in a crisis are those working in the "trenches" day in and day out.

I am still amazed by the indomitable spirit of the people I meet. Generally, as in my mother's case, the patient herself is such an inspiration that she wills others to move forward and do what has to be done. That's what happens in a life threatening situation—we do what is necessary, and we keep fighting. Robert Frost may have put it best: "The best way out is always through."

One of the gifts I received during my journey as a breast cancer advocate was meeting Matt Loscalzo and Jim Zabora, who were both working at Johns Hopkins at the time. When I spoke with them for the first time in the winter of 2000, they expressed a strong desire to work with Men Against Breast Cancer, and right then I knew we had something. Matt and Jim are two of the most gifted and respected people in their field, but more importantly, they are caring human beings whose top priority is the patient's quality of life, including family interaction. As you read this guide, you'll see why Matt is the best at what he does. As a result of meeting him and Jim, I also met Clint Crews, an equally compassionate man who has become an invaluable member of the MABC team.

Another gift I must mention is the honor of meeting and becoming friends with my cofounder, Steve Peck. Steve personifies our message with his personal story of his family's battle against breast cancer. His grace and class are examples we should all live by.

Please know this guide was developed to help you in your unique situation. No guide, and no person, can tell you "the answer" to the problems that breast cancer creates in your relationship and/or family—solving those is something you and she will have to work together to figure out for yourselves. But I have no doubt that if you've picked up this book; you are ready and willing to commit to that task.

I hope that the following advice, information, and encouragement helps you in your battle against breast cancer, just as I hope for health, happiness, and a lot of laughter for you and your family in the future.

—Marc Heyison

Introduction

This is a no-nonsense navigation and survival guide for men who are serious about helping women with breast cancer. If a woman you love has this disease and you want to help her fight it, this is a good place to find out how.

With the right tools, knowledge, skills, and attitude, every man is capable of being extremely helpful in supporting women with breast cancer. This survival guide distills the most important information into key strategies that will give you a better understanding of what she and you are up against.

What this guide *isn't* is a long list of expected social niceties or a series of personal stories. It *is* a highly structured road map, based on many years of practical clinical experience and scientific research, of how a man

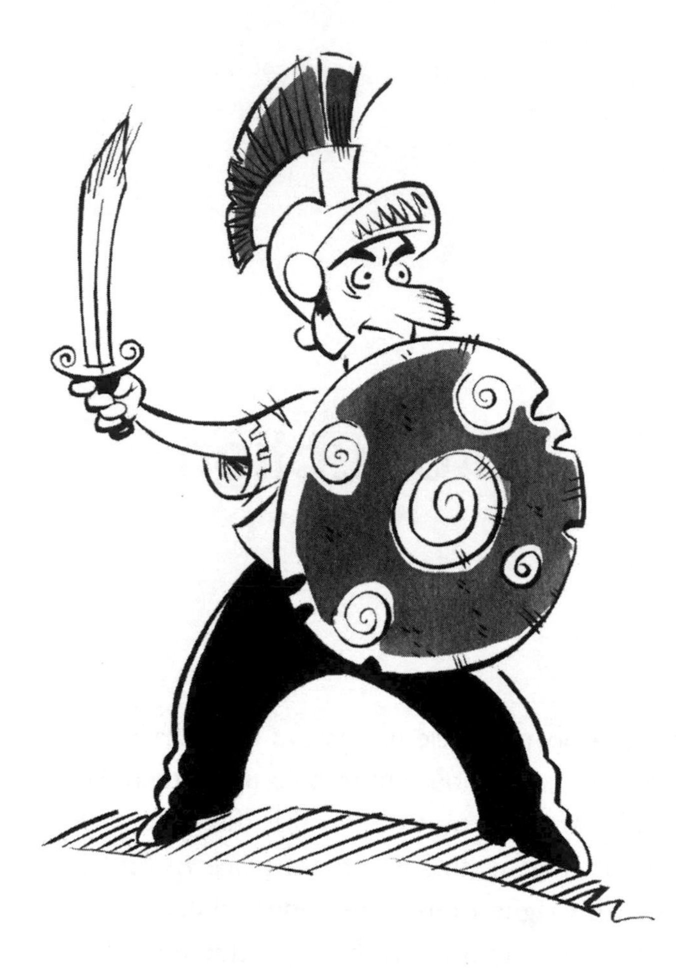

can best help a woman negotiate the many complex problems and disruptions she will encounter in this situation.

Most women with breast cancer welcome support from men as they tackle the difficulties of their illness, and scientific research and clinical experience demonstrate that such support can have a dramatic impact on women's ability to cope. Given the right tools, *you* can make a real difference in the fight against breast cancer.

Choose to be a Courageous and Committed Man

You have a choice: are you going to be helpful, or burdensome? When it comes to a chronic, life-threatening disease like breast cancer, there is no middle ground. This guide will help you choose to be the kind of man who stands strong.

Although the skills you will learn and refine through this guide will help you support the woman with breast cancer, your own life will also be enhanced. You will become a better problem-solver as your creativity, optimism, confidence, and courage increase. The benefits to you, to the woman, and to others in your life who see you taking on this challenge like a man will be extraordinarily rewarding.

The challenge you're facing today is a daunting one, but you can learn to confront it with confidence. After all, we men have been taking on difficult endeavors since the beginning of time. Breast cancer is a serious trial, but it is also an opportunity to prove your love and commitment.

What to Expect From This Guide

In the first Chapter, "Men and Women: Communicating in a Crisis," you will find helpful techniques you can use to bridge the gap between the woman's style of communication and your own. Here you will learn how to set the scene for a discussion, how to signal that you're listening when she speaks, how to share your own feelings, and more. And if you want to know why it's okay to say "What can I do to help?" but not "I understand how you feel," check out the "Say This/Don't Say This" chart on page 22.

You'll need those communication skills when following our problem solving process, called The COPE Model. This ten-step system uses the fundamental tools of Creativity, Optimism, Planning, and Expert information to resolve the complex and often unfamiliar problems that chronic illness can create. You and the woman you love can follow along with Deb and Carlos, and other couples that are dealing with Deb's breast cancer, as they target a problem, gather information, brainstorm creative solutions, and plan their attack.

The "Caregiving for Men" chapter covers all the specific, everyday information you'll need to get through this difficult time, including advice on taking care of her, looking to your own needs, seeking support from your community, and dealing with financial complications. Here you will also find tips on how to cope with non-couple relationships and breast cancer. You will learn how to behave with compassion and sensitivity toward a sister, mother, aunt, niece, or close friend who is sick. You will also learn how to do what is best for any children involved—yours, hers, or both of yours. This chapter also includes a list of danger signs to watch for (like social withdrawal or insomnia) and tells you who to contact if they appear.

Menopause can be confusing to men no matter what the circumstances, but breast cancer often exacerbates the situation. "Menopause: What Men Can Do" will help you understand the changes she's going through so you can navigate them together.

The demands of breast cancer change frequently, which

is why we have a chapter devoted to "Coping with the Phases of Breast Cancer." For each stage of the illness (including diagnosis, treatment, and even the end of life), there is advice for how you can take action, gain knowledge, and provide support during that time. You may want to skip to the section that directly concerns you, but this chapter can also prepare you for what to expect in the future.

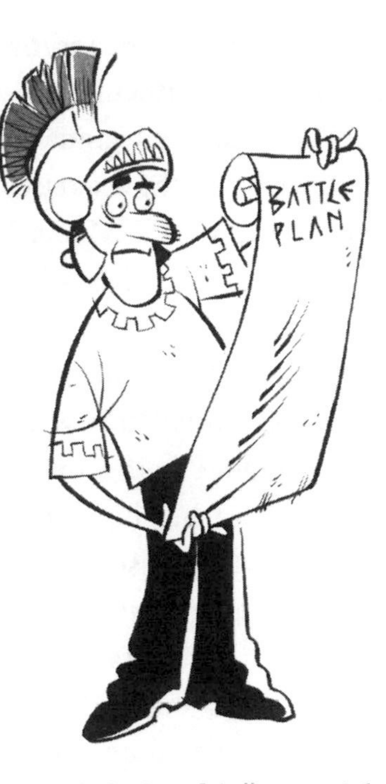

The next chapter deals with "Keeping the Romance in Your Relationship"—a tricky and troubling subject when the woman you love has breast cancer. You will not only learn how to deal with physical complications that arise, but how to keep the romance from fading from your relationship. This chapter teaches you how to talk about intimacy in a constructive, sensitive way that will help the two of you continue to enjoy each other despite her illness.

The final chapter of this book is devoted to "Survivorship." It will help you determine the best ways to help the woman move on. You'll learn how to keep communication open, how to manage and keep tabs on her physical condition, how to help her return to work, and how to deal with uncertainty about her future health and your future as a couple and/or family. This last chapter even addresses the difficult subject of preparing to say goodbye.

For additional guidance or information on any chapter, check out the exercises at the end of each chapter, as well as the COPE Model Worksheet and list of resources in the back of the book.

Be forewarned: although this guide builds on your existing strengths and knowledge, it also demands that you open your mind to new ways of thinking and taking risks. This includes being open to how the woman feels and thinks about her unique experience, even if what she says doesn't make sense to you.

Remember that for a woman with breast cancer, life will never be the same. Even many years after treatment, even if she is cured, her fears, and yours, will linger. This may be harder than you think. Nevertheless, this is your challenge—and your opportunity. You must be her loving, supportive warrior. You will have to make adjustments, think strategically, share emotions, and stay hopeful. You will have to be strong.

It's time to enlist in the fight against breast cancer. You've just taken the first step—and you are needed.

Men and Women: Communicating in a Crisis

Communication is your best weapon in the battle against breast cancer. The deep sense of connection people feel once they know they are heard and understood helps to control fear and creates a sense of strength and direction. It's hard to overestimate how important it is that you're able to talk to the woman you love—about breast cancer, about your feelings, about her feelings, and about your relationship. This section will get you in the right frame of mind to communicate. Here you'll find the preparation and key phrases you'll need to speak effectively.

Men and Women Are More Alike Than Different

There is no war between the sexes, and there never has been. Men and women have done incredible things together throughout the ages. Think about it: we've built homes, raised families, created schools and hospitals. And hopefully, someday very soon, we'll cure breast cancer together.

You've seen shows like *Everybody Loves Raymond*, *The King of Queens*, and *Yes Dear*. To watch these shows, you'd think that men and women are natural enemies. Since the early days of *Jackie Gleason* and *I Love Lucy*, television and the mass media have often made men out to be self-centered and incompetent fools, while women seem to be manipulative demons or sex objects. These disrespectful and insulting stereotypes have been repeated so often that too many men buy into them.

Your job is to remember that often these myths are created solely for profit—at your expense. In reality, individual men and women can have many similarities. Very few sweeping statements can safely be made because every relationship is unique and so are the people involved.

But the Differences *Are* Important!

Although scientific research has clearly demonstrated that the differences between women and men are few compared to the similarities, those differences do exist, and they must be respected.

As you've probably noticed, communication has a way of highlighting the differences between men and women. One of the reasons for this is that some men (though not all) are less than comfortable talking about their emotional concerns and fears. Many women, on the other hand, find it very comforting to talk openly about things that may be upsetting, like the impact of treatments, physical changes, loss of a job, or fears that the treatments won't work.

When women find themselves in difficult situations, few prefer to act as if there is nothing wrong. Women feel safer and more secure when they share their fears and vunerabilities; generally, men do not. This means that women with breast cancer need to talk about their experiences and feelings. However, they are often more comfortable taking care of others and don't want to feel like a burden to loved ones. This can create an internal conflict for those women.

Men tend to avoid *interpersonal emotional content* because they are taught from a young age to ignore their emotions. They are expected to be *men*, and not to behave "like girls." It is also probably true that men aren't genetically programmed to be as connected to their emotions as women are. So when you add societal pressure to genetic predisposition, it's easy to understand men's frustration when they are suddenly expected to act in ways that don't come naturally and, in fact, were discouraged earlier in life.

What men need to realize is that emotions don't have to be inconvenient or embarrassing. Properly focused and directed, they can actually be the fuel that drives them to succeed. Men who learn to harness their emotions are better able to motivate themselves and connect to others. They're more fully alive.

Men don't like talking about situations that make them feel powerless. They don't want to think about the fact that they can't solve a loved one's problems. This fear of powerlessness is limiting, and when dealing with an emotionally-charged situation like a loved one's illness, it can be devastating. How can you defeat breast cancer if you can't even make yourself talk about it?

The problem is that many men don't see "connecting" through talking as doing something concrete to help. But it is. Consider what we've just said about a woman's need to communicate. It might not always make sense to you, but talking to a woman about her feelings is one of the most important ways you can help her feel connected and safe. You can't cure cancer, but you *can* make her feel better by learning to communicate.

Mission-Based vs. Process-Based Behavior

"Mission-based" and "process-based" are two styles of behavior that influence the way people communicate. As you're reading, it might sound like the two styles describe men and women, especially given the generalities we've just outlined. But in reality, you're likely to find that you and the woman you love each have some mission-based and some process-based characteristics. Neither style is definitively male or female.

Mission-Based Behavior

Mission-based people are very good at getting things done. They focus on the next step, the plan of action, the practical thing to do. The process (what happens along the way while working toward a goal) is not what matters most to mission-based people. They tend to prize the result rather than the effort, and are particularly interested in their individual contribution. They do not show their weaknesses because to the mission-based person, this seems dangerous.

When mission-based people feel stressed, they focus on exactly what needs to be done next to accomplish the mission. For the most part, they avoid the emotional side of things because they see it as a distraction from the goal at hand. Emotions can't be solved or fixed, and they don't always make sense. Although mission-based people may be very committed to others, they are less likely to talk openly about their love, fears, or concerns.

Mission-based people cope well when they can do something to make things better—and not so well when they can't. Emotional, social, and physical withdrawal is common in mission-based individuals when they feel stressed or powerless. This can also upset those around them. For mission-based men, the ultimate act of courage is saying to the women they love, "There is nothing we can't talk about and face together."

Process-Based Behavior

Process-based people are very good at maintaining relationships and doing multiple things at once. They are sensitive to their environment, especially in family life. Communication and connection are very important to them. They like to share an experience as it's happening and discuss it afterwards. A blow-by-blow account of an event is almost as important as the event's outcome.

To show vulnerability, for the process-based person, is to engage others and to lessen the sense of fear. Sharing

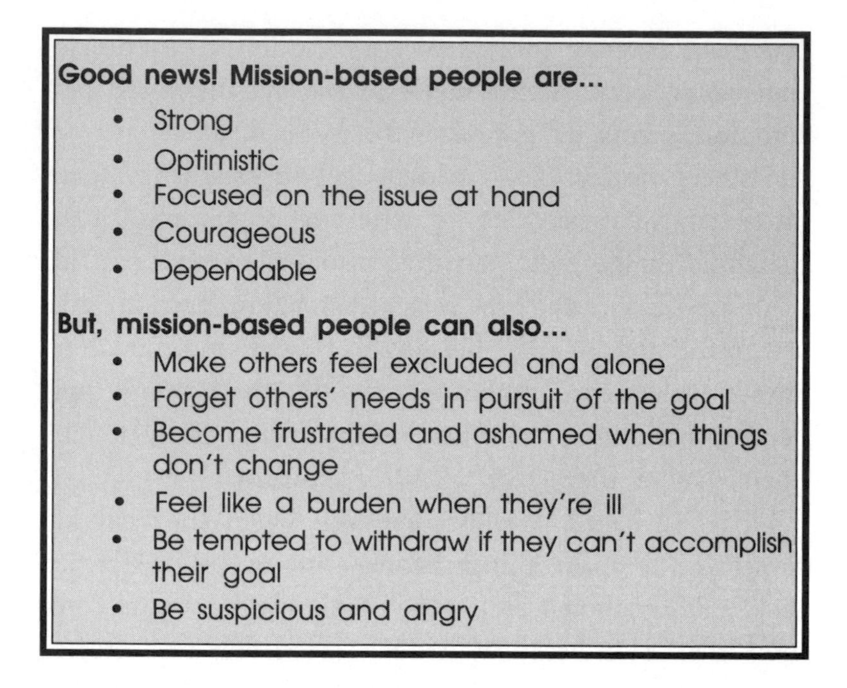

Good news! Mission-based people are...

- Strong
- Optimistic
- Focused on the issue at hand
- Courageous
- Dependable

But, mission-based people can also...

- Make others feel excluded and alone
- Forget others' needs in pursuit of the goal
- Become frustrated and ashamed when things don't change
- Feel like a burden when they're ill
- Be tempted to withdraw if they can't accomplish their goal
- Be suspicious and angry

weakness makes them feel stronger because they are allied with others (this is sometimes called "circling the wagons"). Process-based people value social and personal interaction and working together. Regardless of how unpleasant or scary an experience may be, they gain a deep sense of connection by sharing it with others. For example, they might openly share feelings about their illness, or a loved one's, with someone they hardly know. A mission-based person will only share that kind of information if the benefit to the outcome is obvious.

Clearly, the mission-based and process-based styles of behavior are extreme types, but they can help you understand how you and others manage problems. Nothing is quite as upsetting as being told that the way you handle problems is wrong or doesn't make sense. Learning the reasoning behind others' behavior can help you avoid that insensitivity.

For example, a man has noticed a communication problem in his relationship, so instead of giving up or trying to guess what she wants, he asks her about it:

"Lately you've been telling me how scared you feel about all the things that can go wrong because of breast cancer. I've been listing ideas for what we could do, but you never take my suggestions. I feel like you haven't been hearing me. I care about you and I don't want to bother you. Would it be helpful if I just listened? Or is there something you need to hear from me?"

People are different, which is what makes life so wonderful and so challenging. It takes a lot of cooperation and courage to balance the needs of two people, and recognizing your own (and your partner's) communication style and working to overcome its limitations is the first step.

Good news! Process-based people are...

- Nurturing
- Communicative
- Sensitive to others' distress
- Able to tolerate powerlessness and hopelessness
- Often the emotional center of a family

But, process-based people can also...

- Be overly sensitive to rejection
- Worry too much about isolation and abandonment
- Exhaust themselves supporting others
- Often feel guilty, anxious, and depressed

Something to Think About

"Never assume" is the first and most important rule of communication. Remind yourself of this each and every time you start a conversation with the woman you love.

Consider what she's dealing with. Even if her prognosis for recovery is excellent, she is still confronting an uncertain future. Her life will never be the same. She is constantly concerned about the many possible consequences of her illness such as increased risk to children, reoccurrence of the cancer side affects of treatments, etc. Those worries never go away.

No matter how close you two are, she is the one facing the physical reality of breast cancer, not you. The situation may be very tough for you, too, but that doesn't automatically mean you'll know how she feels or what she needs.

Don't start by telling her what you think she needs to fix. If you're going to bring up a problem, start with a breast cancer-related problem that *you* want to work on. For example, you might want to learn how to control your anger. Self-awareness will make you both feel more comfortable and less threatened. Besides, choosing your own problem to work on will make you more invested in reaching a positive outcome—and when she's ready, the same will apply to her. Just let her bring up her problems in her own time, and don't try to speed things up.

Ready, Set, Talk

How to Set the Scene

When you sit down to talk, first make sure that you

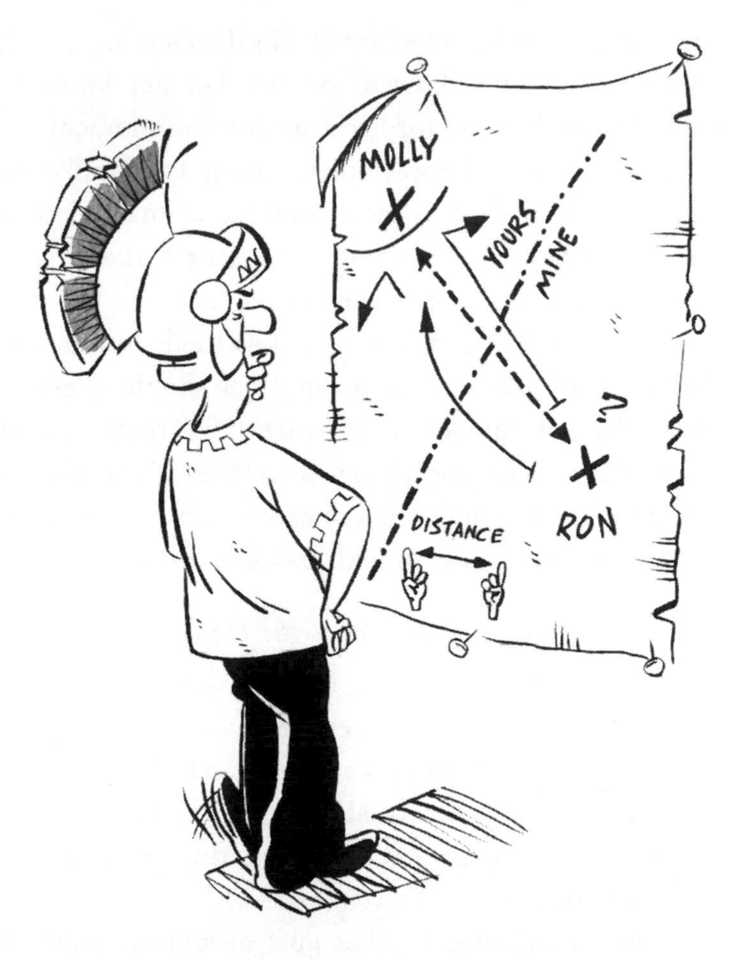

both have enough time to devote to a conversation. Generally, it takes about ten to fifteen minutes of talking openly and honestly before a problem surfaces. (Note: If you don't think you have any specific problems to work on, then one or both of you is probably not being honest.)

Choose a private, safe place to start your conversation, somewhere where you both feel comfortable and you're unlikely to be interrupted. No distractions or interruptions should be allowed, period. Let her know that talking to her is your top priority for the moment.

Pay attention to the way you're sitting, too. Unlike men, who may avoid face-to-face contact, women generally prefer it. They see it as a sign of closeness and trust. Sit where you can make eye contact.

Another thing: don't forget (or be afraid) to touch her! Take her hand, put an arm around her shoulder, give her a hug. Physical contact is extremely important to a sick person. She is very susceptible to feelings of isolation and abandonment. As long as you're gentle, touching will make both of you feel more united and less alone.

How to Say the Right Thing

- Be honest. Don't just tell the woman what you think she wants to hear, because she knows you and she'll probably be able to tell. Don't risk undermining her trust. Hiding the truth from her will only come across as deceitful or condescending.
- Be courageous. It takes guts to address topics like the way your sex life has changed or the possibility of her death, but at some point you'll have to do it. Prepare yourself so that you'll be ready to talk about the hard stuff whenever she's ready.
- Be delicate. Yes, talk about how you honestly feel and talk about the hard topics. But remember also that she's in a fragile state of mind. Try to be as tactful as possible. Keep in mind that your phras-

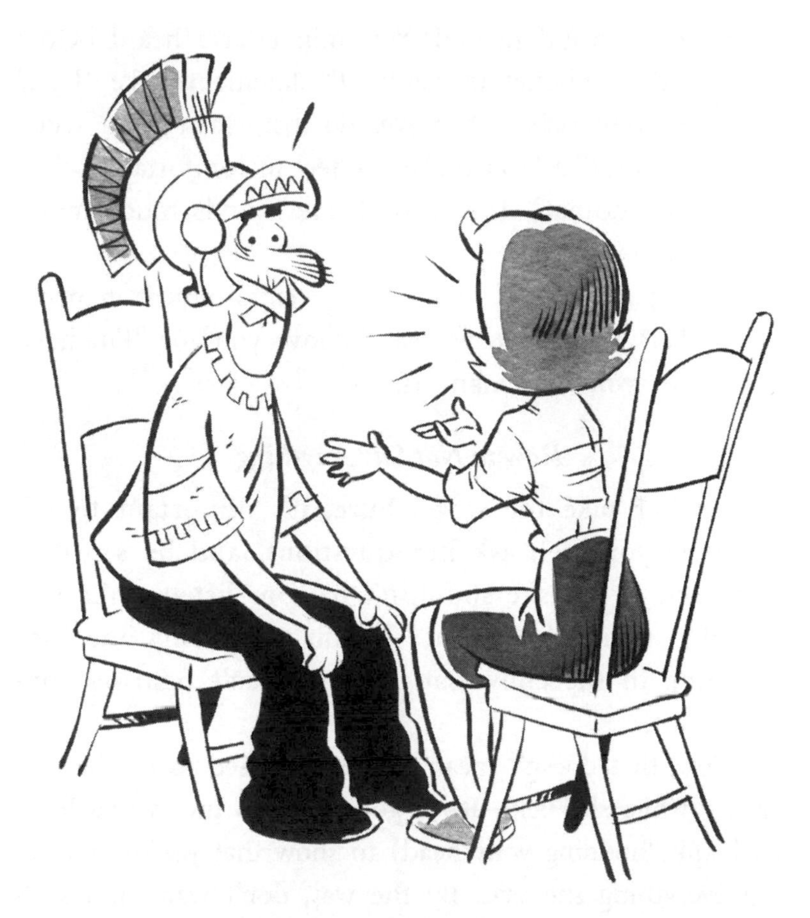

ing can make a huge difference. (For examples, see the chart on page 22.)

- Be supportive. This doesn't mean agreeing with everything she says. It does mean not debating or second-guessing her. She is the best authority on her own personal experience. Remember, even if the conversation isn't going smoothly, stay committed to it—just as you are to your relationship.

- Be non-judgmental. You might have heard before that it's better to make "I" statements, like "I feel uncomfortable when you do that," than "you" statements, like "You make me feel uncomfortable when you dothat." The second one sounds much more accusatory.
- Repeat yourself. Women like reinforcement, remember? You can never say "I love you" or "I'm here for you" too many times.

How to Not Say Anything

Let her take the stage. Sure, it's important to tell her how you feel, ask her questions, and be sensitive and honest. But she shouldn't have to listen while you verbally "figure things out." If you're the only one contributing to the conversation, you aren't figuring anything out.

Now, that doesn't mean you're supposed to sit there in silence while she talks. It's a good idea to give visual feedback (like nodding your head) to show that you're processing everything she says. By the way, don't wait until she's finished and then launch off on a new topic. Listen carefully so that you can respond directly to something she said or at least relate her words to something you'd like to talk about. Remember, she doesn't expect you to fix her problems, just to share her fears so she's not alone.

One time when it's okay to sit in silence is when you've just asked the woman you love a hard question and she seems to be sorting out her feelings and thinking about a reply. In this case, it's better to just wait. It might seem like a lifetime, but it's not unusual for thirty seconds or even a full minute to pass.

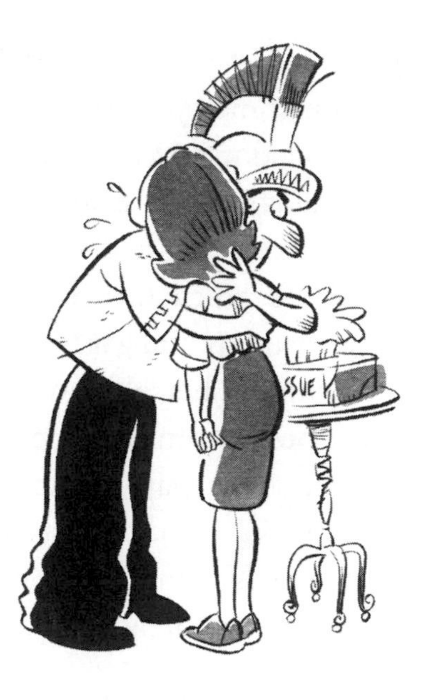

What To Do If...

...she starts to cry, and you don't know why.

You've been a guy long enough to know that when a woman cries, it doesn't necessarily mean something bad has happened. It might be nothing in particular, or even something good. A woman with breast cancer is emotionally vulnerable, so any type of emotion (sadness, happiness, fear, gratitude) can overwhelm her and lead to tears. Remember that your behavior isn't necessarily the cause. She's got a lot on her plate right now, so the crying might have nothing to do with you. Don't jump to conclusions.

Your job, as a man? Don't panic! Her tears won't kill either of you, so don't become frantic trying to stop them. First, hold her (if she'll let you) and wait for her to calm down. Then ask her why she's crying and whether she's still upset. Don't be afraid that you're "supposed to already know," even if she says so. You're not a mind-reader, and guessing is a dangerous game. Ask. Gently. Remember that the emotional content about the interaction is much more important than the actual words you use.

...you get angry at her.

Sometimes you just won't get it. You're not a woman and you don't have breast cancer, so it's likely that you won't always be able to relate. But if your frustration gets the better of you and you become angry, that's a problem.

If and when this happens, your first concern should be to focus your anger toward the situation and away from the woman herself. So maybe she's being irrational, unresponsive, combative, or whatever. Wouldn't you sometimes feel that way, too, in her situation? Never forget that the woman's behavior is constantly impacted by her disease, and is sometimes out of her control. Take a deep breath or go for a walk until you feel under control.

...she gets angry at you.

Give her time to figure out why she's angry. She might not even know why herself. If her response seems irrational or unfair, try not to be offended. It could be that she's looking for somebody to blame and you're a convenient punching bag for the moment. You may be the only person in her life right now with whom she can safely and openly share her frustrations. Cancer is faceless; she can't pin it down and yell at it. If it does seem that she just feels like yelling (which we all do sometimes), try to stay calm and be understanding. *Don't* respond in kind. Wait until she is less upset and then ask her to talk about what just happened.

...she won't talk to you.

It takes two to untangle a problem in any relationship,

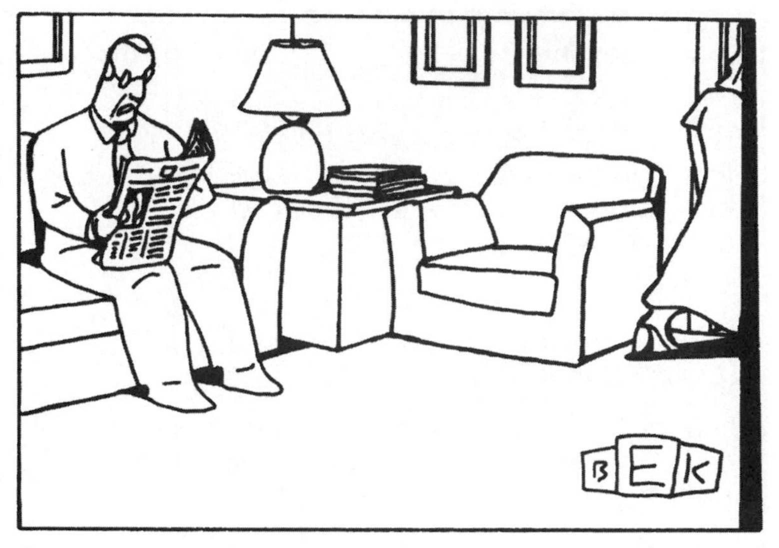

"Don't walk away from me while I'm not paying any attention to you."

so if she's unwilling to participate, there isn't much you can do. This will take a judgment call on your part. Is it just a passing mood? Does she need time to sort out her feelings? Or will you need to coax her into a conversation? If she's really resistant, your best bet is to lay your cards on the table: "I'd really like to hear how you're feeling, but I don't want to bug you if you need space. Please come to me as soon as you feel like talking." Keep asking periodically so she's sure you haven't forgotten. If she hasn't opened up in a long time and seems depressed, it might be best if she spoke to a counselor.

...she keeps repeating herself.

Here's something we guys really don't understand. Why do women want to go over the same conversational territory again and again—in excruciating detail? Remember

Say This	Don't Say This
"I love you." These are the most important words you can say—over and over.	*"I agree with you."* It's a conversation-stopper. Tell her why.
"I think I heard you say (blank), is that right?" Repeat back what she's told you to show that you were listening.	*"I understand how you feel."* This can sound to the woman like a refusal to discuss the issue.
"I don't understand, can you explain that?" It's okay to admit it!	*"If you would just..."* Don't try to be Mr. Fix-It. She'll resent it, and it won't help.
"What can I do to help?" You won't know unless you ask.	*"There's nothing to be afraid of."* This seems like a dismissal of her fears. Besides, you both know it isn't true.
"How do you feel about..." This invites her to speak and shows that you care.	*"It's all for the best."* Cancer is never for the best, and you don't have to pretend it is.

that talking is what makes a woman feel connected to others, and that she needs connection now on a very regular basis. There might not be anything new to talk about, but that doesn't mean she doesn't need to discuss something. There is nothing pathological about needing to share a traumatic experience, even repeatedly. So have a seat and get ready to listen one more time.

Dealing with Verbal Conflicts

Men are particularly sensitive to being disrespected by others. Because of this, it is not easy for men to ignore unfair treatment. But as you know, in any long-lasting relationship there are bound to be times when feelings get hurt.

Although it's usually healthy to discuss hurt feelings, sometimes the best solution is to take ten deep breaths and just forget about it. People bug each other sometimes, and that's okay. It's not worth the effort of getting angry at every minor disagreement, especially when both of you are going through a stressful time. Stress can cause chemical changes in the brain that make people act totally out of character. Try to be patient and supportive, and time will help to heal the wounds. Most often, as the stress level declines, so will the unpleasant behavior.

However, verbal abuse is never okay. If you think the situation is escalating and that one or both of you is going over-the-top, leave the room immediately. You may need to wait a few hours or a day before you (gently) try to talk about what happened. If verbal abuse becomes a pattern, reach out for professional help.

Issue	Problem
Something that you care about but does not directly impact the essential part of your life in a meaningful way. You can live with it.	*Something that you care about that* does *impact you personally and has to be managed or your life will not work as well.*
My car is filthy and has mice	My car has a broken axel and I am on the highway with my family
World hunger	My family is hungry
The doctor is a cold fish	The doctor does not give us the information we need to make informed decisions
Our children are sad because their mom is ill	Our children see that their mom is ill but we are "protecting" them by not telling them what is happening
47 million Americans do not have health insurance and twice as many are grossly under-insured	We have lost our health insurance and cannot pay our bills

Sometimes a few brief counseling sessions to discuss the conflict with a social worker or a psychologist can be all you need to get back on track. All reputable hospitals and many physician offices have trained and licensed mental health professionals (either social workers, psychologists, psychiatrists) readily available to help support patients and their family members. So if you're in doubt, reach out for help—the sooner, the better.

Remember, meeting with a mental health professional doesn't mean you've failed. In fact, it shows that you are willing to do whatever it takes to improve your communication skills and defeat breast cancer. Try the Resources listed in the back of this book to find a counselor. You'll be glad you did, and so will the rest of your family.

Issues are Not Problems

Serious illness has a way of focusing how we think. It also helps us realize what really matters. Knowing how to prioritize and to best invest your resources (money, energy, love, time, etc.) is essential to making conscious choices about what matters to you most. One way to do this is to know the difference between an *issue* and a *problem*, as outlined on the previous page.

An issue is something that you may care or feel strongly about but is not essential to your daily life. Something that interferes with your daily life and is important to manage is a problem, not an issue.

When considering where to put your resources, it is important that your thinking be very clear. Remember, you are the one your family looks to for confidence, honesty, and guidance. No one expects you to know the answers, but you *are* expected to get everyone focused on what matters most.

The COPE Model can be especially helpful if you involve your family in the problem-solving process. Joint action teaches others how to effectively solve problems, creates a sense of meaningful activity, and deepens your family connection. Now is the time to focus on real problems that: (1) matter most to you and your family today, (2) you can have some influence over, and (3) will result in a direct benefit to you and your family.

The COPE Model of Problem Solving

Dealing with cancer is an emotional and stressful experience. It causes a lot of stress, and that can make everyone involved pretty hard to be around. The difficulty of the situation will exaggerate any differences between the way you cope with stress and the way the woman chooses to cope—and there *will* be differences. But in a way, the situation also creates an opportunity. This is your chance to prove your commitment to this woman and learn what it means to be a courageous man.

The COPE Model* is a problem-solving system that uses the fundamental building blocks of *Creativity*, *Optimism*, *Planning*, and *Expert information* to form a list of

---

The COPE Model theory was originally developed by Dr. Peter Houts:
Houts, PS. (Ed.) *Home Care Guide for Cancer.* American College of Surgeons, 1994.

step-by-step instructions. Following these instructions is a fast and proven way for you and the woman you love to resolve many of the problems you are facing.

Remember to take your time. Rushing through any process usually leads to bad decisions and poor results, and in this case, your results are crucial. The last thing you want is to make things harder for the woman.

Before you try out the COPE Model, it is important to make sure that the two of you are both committed to

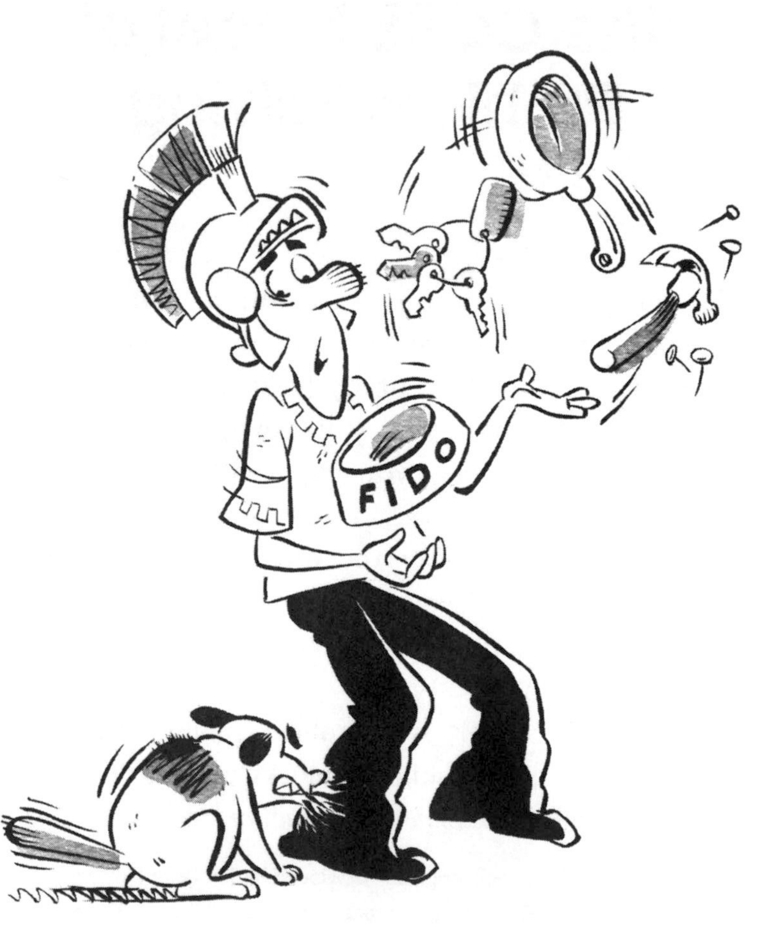

following it. You won't solve anything if one partner is pushing the other to participate or making all the decisions. The COPE Model will work best if you are in this together.

The COPE model is a powerful tool to use when solving complex problems. Using Creativity, Optimism, Planning, and Expert Information will enable your family to work as a team to feel more connected, to be more efficient, and to have a sense of meaningful direction that can control fear and minimize depression. But, as is all too often the reality in life, the COPE model demands that you are a bit flexible and start backwards, beginning with the E in Expert Information. We all know that faulty information, it can be disastrous. So when deciding to be a wise and courageous man it is important to get the cold brutal facts first!

The Fundamentals of COPE

Creativity You already know that in relationships, as in life, problems often aren't solved on the first try. That means you'll need to get creative to find new and better solutions. You might think that you aren't a very creative person, but this kind of creativity is a skill that can be learned. All you have to do is put in the effort.

Optimism If you don't think you can make things better, you won't. Maintaining a positive outlook is essential, not only while working with the COPE Model, but throughout your battle with breast cancer. Like creativity, optimism might seem like a personality trait you either have

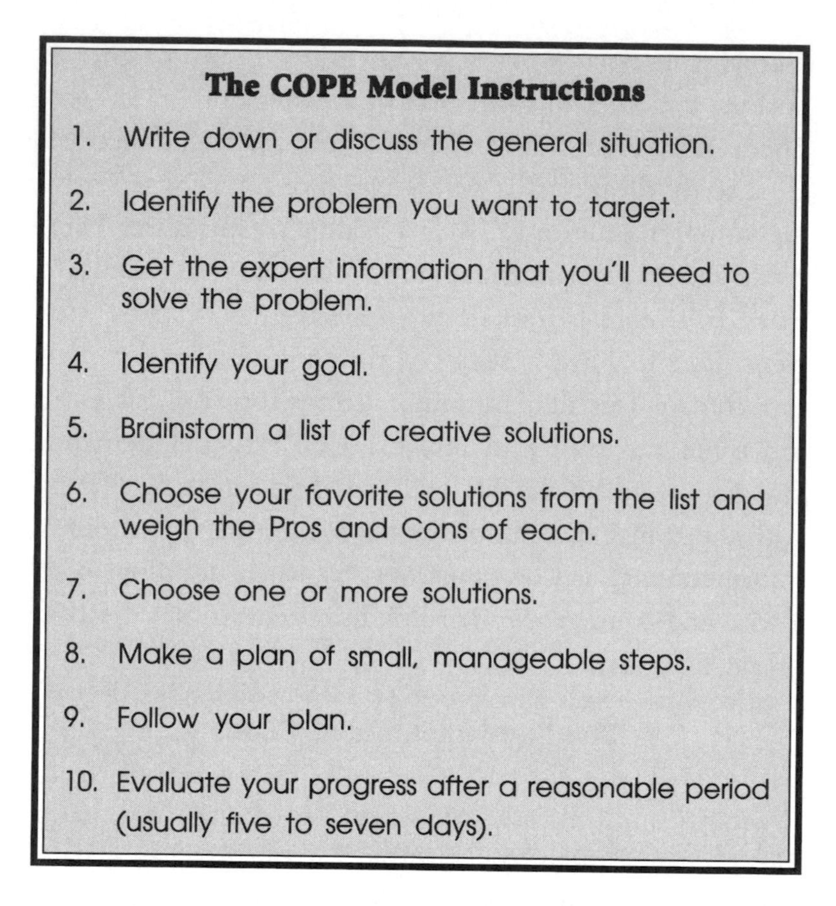

The COPE Model Instructions

1. Write down or discuss the general situation.
2. Identify the problem you want to target.
3. Get the expert information that you'll need to solve the problem.
4. Identify your goal.
5. Brainstorm a list of creative solutions.
6. Choose your favorite solutions from the list and weigh the Pros and Cons of each.
7. Choose one or more solutions.
8. Make a plan of small, manageable steps.
9. Follow your plan.
10. Evaluate your progress after a reasonable period (usually five to seven days).

or don't have. But the truth is, your attitude is a choice. Decide right now that your glass is half full.

Planning Creativity and optimism are all well and good, but without a plan (and the guts to execute it), you won't get far. This is the practical part. You'll need to use the knowledge you've gained from past experiences to determine the course of action that is most likely to succeed.

Expert information It is almost impossible to know how

to effectively manage a situation without accurate medical information. Maybe some of the problems you are having with the woman you love are rooted in biological changes caused by her illness. (In fact, many probably are.) Good expert information can also prevent confusion. For example, it's pretty important to know that when looking for cancer "negative test results" means good news for a cancer patient.

Step 1: Write down or discuss the general situation.

Before you start, you and the woman you love need to express how you both are feeling. This doesn't mean you have to agree on who's wrong and who's right, or who needs to do what. Just write out the general situation at this point in your breast cancer battle. And don't worry if there seems to be lots of problems tangled together—you'll sort it out later.

Take the situation below. It may sound familiar. Women report that men tend to be very helpful when the diagnosis is new. Men are very good at helping women be optimistic, finding a physician, getting back and forth to treatments, etc. When the mission is clear, men do very well. Women very much appreciate these extremely helpful functions. However, women also report that as treatment ends and the initial crisis of the new diagnosis and treatment passes, women need something very different from men. For men, this can be very confusing.

Women now need you to shift from Mission Mode to Process Mode. In Mission Mode, the most important thing is to get the mission accomplished, while in Process Mode,

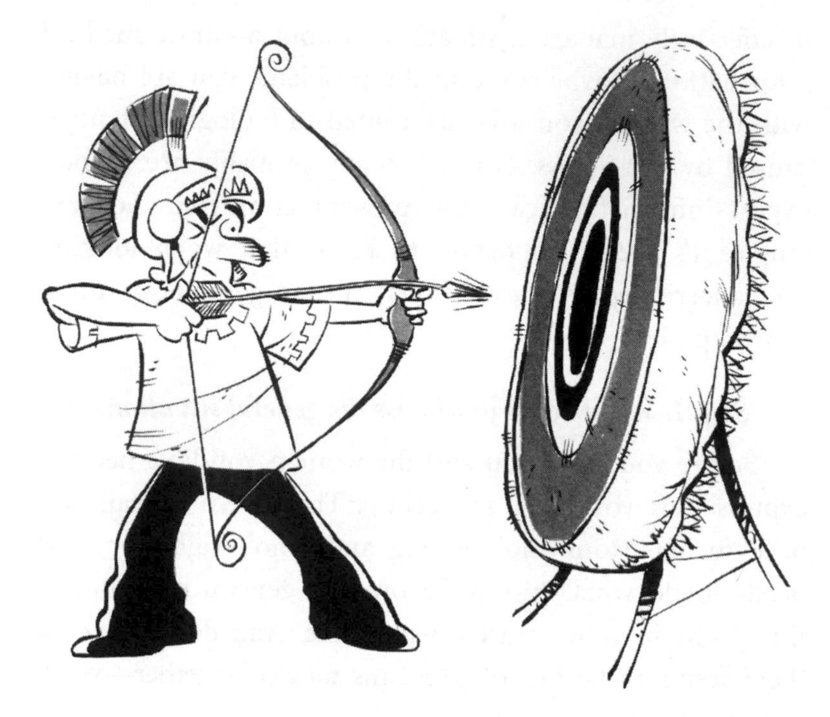

the higher value is placed on the relationship—feeling deeply connected to other human beings. This is time for assessing the damage and healing.

Deb and Carlos have been married for twenty-five years and have had a happy marriage. Three months ago, Deb had a mastectomy. When Deb first found out that she had breast cancer she was amazed and grateful at how helpful Carlos was throughout this entire period. Carlos told Deb that she should have expected no less and that he loved her very much and would always be there for her. Now that the immediate crisis is over, Deb says that the reality of what the cancer did to her and the loss of her breast has hit her like the "Empire State Building falling on her." Deb says, "I am no longer who I was. I could have died." Carlos tries to support Deb by telling her not to dwell on it. He is very optimistic, but this only upsets Deb. For the first time in twenty-five years, Deb and Carlos are having serious marital conflicts. Carlos feels like he can do nothing right and is withdrawing.

Step 2: Identify the problem you want to target.

You've established how you both feel and the negative effects you are suffering. Now you must try and boil down the situation to something tangible and solvable. Choose problems that are quite specific, such as talking about the illness with family members, getting information from the doctor, managing pain or fatigue, or coping with depression. If the problem is not clearly defined, it is too hard to measure when and how it has improved. If this happens, you'll get frustrated and be much less likely to continue with the process. You will feel even worse than when you started.

The problem you highlight should also have energy—it should have *juice!* That means it should create just enough emotion so that you care about solving or managing it, but not so much emotion that you feel overwhelmed by feelings. Also, beware of problems that have been going on for a long time and are not related to the situation at hand. Long-standing marital problems or past hurts are generally best handled by a professional counselor.

To sum up, these are the criteria you'll want to make sure your problem meets:

- The problem is clearly defined and solvable.
- The problem is related to the effects of breast cancer and isn't left over from previous marital troubles.
- You are highly motivated to work on this specific problem now.
- The changes in the problem can be measured so you'll be able to tell when things are getting better.
- The difficulty of the problem is proportionate to your skill level in using the COPE Model.

After you get good at using the COPE Model you can work on harder problems, but for now, try to set yourself up to succeed. Start small and persevere!

One more note: make sure the words you use to describe the problem are non-judgmental. For example, don't say, "Deb keeps trying to dwell on her pain, while Carlos wants to focus on the future and think positively." You also shouldn't say, "Deb wants to tell Carlos how she is feeling, while Carlos doesn't want to talk about it."

These might sound like your own first interpretations of your problem, but they are also unfair and antagonistic. Keep in mind that the two of you are on the same team. Acknowledge that you both want to make things better by using balanced language and staying away from emotionally charged phrases:

Deb would like to communicate her feelings of fear and depression, while Carlos thinks it would be best to move on and stop focusing on all the bad things caused by the cancer.

Step 3: Get the expert information that you'll need to solve the problem.

A woman experiences many physical changes following a mastectomy, and understanding them will help you and the woman you love better understand her disease and each other. Obviously, if the changes mean the cancer has returned, then a medical assessment is crucial. But unpleasant effects like pain, insomnia, and fatigue can also influence the woman's behavior and feelings about your relationship. If the woman's physical discomfort can be bettter managed or eliminated, and if she can be told that her pain is *not* a recurrence of breast cancer, there will be much less stress for both of you.

First, locate your sources of information. Your physician can give you medical advice, and nurses will also be able to help you with common physical symptoms. For information about mental health and coping with stress, consult a social worker, psychologist or psychiatrist. Having the correct information will help ensure that your eventual plan to solve the problem will target the right issues. If you and the woman try to communicate based on assumptions and guesses at each other's motivations, you'll be setting yourselves up to fail. Neither of you is a mind reader!

Here are some questions that Deb and Carlos could ask to help them better deal with their own feelings and understand the other's:

- What are the chances of Deb's cancer returning?

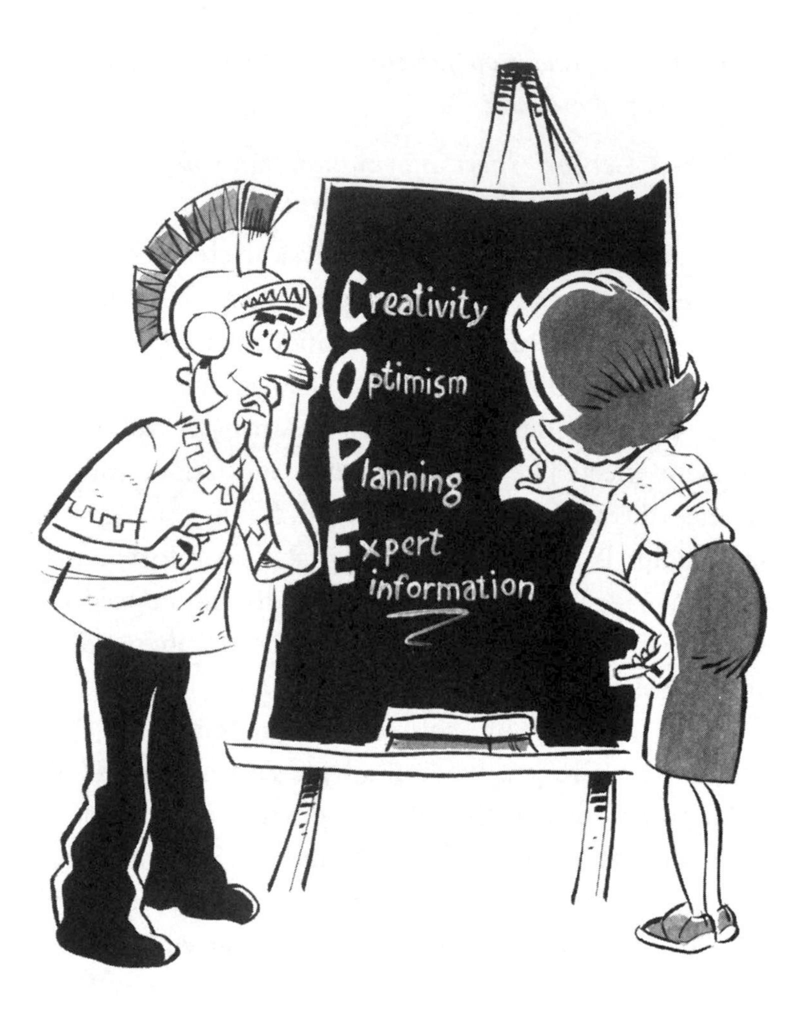

- Why do cancer patients become depressed even after successful treatment?
- Does Carlos run any risk of depression if he thinks about cancer all the time?
- How can depression be treated?
- Can fears be "talked out," or does dwelling on them typically make them worse?

These questions may not yield conclusive answers. The answers might not even be very reassuring. Nevertheless, in the battle against breast cancer, you need to be prepared. Even something as simple as making sure you understand the relevant terminology can make a big difference.

Step 4: Identify your goal.

This step could be trickier than it sounds. You know that you both want to be happier with yourselves and with each other, but if you have conflicting interests, it can be hard to settle on an ideal outcome. Choose a goal that addresses both partners' needs. Also, make sure it's realistic. The ordeal of breast cancer has already taught you that there are no magic solutions. Still, that's no reason things can't get much, much better. (This is where *Optimism* comes in.)

Deb and Carlos' goal is to enable Deb to express her concerns to Carlos without Carlos feeling that they are unnecessarily rehashing the pain of breast cancer.

Step 5: Brainstorm a list of creative solutions.

The primary tool of *Creativity* is brainstorming, although there are lots of other creative ways to achieve your goals. Both of you should contribute to a long list of possible activities or strategies that you think might help you solve the problem. Remember, brainstorming is intended to create as many varied solutions as possible, so make sure to withhold judgment during this step. Right now, anything goes.

Some people are turned off by the idea of "brainstorming." It's corny, for one. Some also have a hard time controlling knee-jerk negative reactions to others' new ideas. It's easy to quickly dismiss them or make excuses. Maybe you can manage all the problems in your own life, but when it comes to relationships with other people, it is always helpful to get community input – even if that community is just you and the woman. Try to be open and go with the flow.

Here's where *Optimism*—even fake optimism—can be especially effective. Many people are surprised to find that even just acting like they feel optimistic can make new solutions suddenly appear. This isn't magic. Hope and creativity tend to feed off each other. A positive attitude often yields good ideas, just as one good idea can inspire a more hopeful attitude.

Here are some ideas that Deb and Carlos might come up with (which doesn't mean they're all good ones, of course!):

- Write letters to each other once a week telling each other how they feel
- Deb lists all of the things she is worried about and she and Carlos discuss them
- See a marital counselor together
- Go on a vacation together
- Plan more intimate time
- Schedule twenty minutes every day for Deb to share her emotional concerns, whether realistic or not, while Carlos listens supportively
- Take some time apart
- Deb shares her concerns with other family members and her friends more often
- Deb and Carlos get drunk and have a good long cry together

SOLUTION	PROS	CONS
Deb and Carlos write letters to each other about how they feel.	It will be a nice change of pace from talking in circles. They can take their time and not get upset or angry. They'll get equal time to express themselves.	Carlos hates writing. After the letters, what will really change?
Go on a vacation together.	No stress from jobs and social life to make things worse. Both need to catch up on sleep. Deb might be able to get her mind off breast cancer.	They might get sick of each other. Logistical problems can make vacations stressful. Money is tight. Deb might spoil activities with bad moods.
Get drunk and cry together.	When this has worked before, they have felt very close.	If they start an argument while drunk, they won't be able to reason clearly. Deb gets drunk faster, hangovers will make them crabby the next day.
Take time apart.	Absence makes the heart grow fonder. Carlos will get a break from breast cancer.	Carlos will worry about Deb. They won't communicate. Deb will feel abandoned.
Deb shares her concerns with other family members and friends.	Deb will be able to express her concerns as often as she likes without always involving Carlos. Deb will feel like she has stronger support and more supporters. Carlos won't feel as guilty if he doesn't want to talk.	Deb will feel she is not being totally open with Carlos.

- Deb reminds herself regularly that she is lucky to be alive
- Speak with their spiritual adviser
- Deb uses art therapies like painting, music, sing ing, sculpture as ways to express herself individually
- Volunteer together at a hospital or shelter
- Take dancing lessons together

Step 6: Choose your favorite solutions from the list and weigh the pros and cons of each.

Once you have generated a sizeable list of creative solutions while withholding judgment, put your "wisdom hat" back on to make some meaningful decisions. Select several ideas that you both support. Then make a table with columns for the pros (possible positive outcomes) and cons (possible negative outcomes) of each idea.

Step 7: Choose one or more solutions.

When you're choosing which solution or solutions to try, don't pick based on the number of Pros and Cons you've generated. Some Cons can outweigh all the positives of an idea, and vice versa. Choose carefully.

Here is what Deb and Carlos might decide:

They decide *not* to write letters. Since Carlos hates writing, it would just feel like a punishment to him.

They decide to take a vacation together. They could really use some time away from the stresses of daily life, and this way Carlos won't feel distracted when Deb wants to talk. To make sure the trip isn't soured if/when Deb feels too depressed to join in activities, they will make it a relaxed vacation with nothing scheduled.

They decide *not* to take time apart. They'll only think about each other more.

They decide *not* to get drunk and cry together. Too many things can go wrong.

They decide Deb should share her concerns with other family members and friends. Carlos won't carry the full burden of listening to her concerns many times over, while Deb will feel happy to make things easier for Carlos and more secure knowing that she has a wide base of support. To keep communication between Deb and Carlos open, Deb will continue to tell him how she feels, just not as often.

Step 8: Make a plan of small, manageable steps.

Your plan probably won't succeed all at once. At the very least you'll have to do some practical preparation. *Planning* is important because once you know what to do, you'll have no excuse not to do it. Also, remember that you are most likely to succeed in your plan of action if your steps are small, at least at first.

Solution #1: They take a vacation together

1. Make a budget for the whole trip.
2. Pick a beach or lake to visit.
3. Check Deb and Carlos' schedules and decide when to go.
4. Check prices, then decide whether to stay in a hotel or rental home.
5. Check flight prices, then decide whether to drive or fly.
6. Schedule the flight OR take the car for a tune-up.
7. Make accommodation reservations.

8. Hire dog sitter.
9. Pack.

Rules for Solution #1

- No laptops or paperwork
- No scheduled activities
- Try to limit discussions of breast cancer to evening talks
- If an issue comes up, work it out then and there—there's lots of time
- Get intimate during mornings or daytime to shake up the usual routine

Solution #2: Deb shares her concerns with others

1. With Carlos' input, Deb decides on two or three "support" people she trusts.
2. Deb calls each new support and asks if they are willing to take time to talk with her when she needs it, making sure they understand the situation.
3. The next time Deb feels she needs to talk, she considers whether this is something she has already discussed with Carlos.
4. She considers the urgency of her own needs.
5. If that urgency is not too great, she considers Carlos' current mood and availability.
6. If the situation is right, she calls her other support until somebody is available to talk with her.
7. Later, when the time is right, she tells Carlos that she spoke to another support and whether the conversation was helpful.
8. If it wasn't, Deb and Carlos then have their own discussion.

Rules for Solution #2

- If Deb is feeling very depressed or upset, she must tell Carlos
- If Deb is in physical pain, she must tell Carlos
- Carlos must respect the privacy of Deb's interactions with her other supporters

Step 9: Follow your plan. Right now!

Sounds simple, right? But you're likely to find that doing what you say you'll do is the most challenging part of all—kind of like that time you promised to empty the dishwasher every night. Stick with it if you want to see results.

On the other hand, if you find that your plan is stressing you out or is just plain too hard, it's time to get together and revise it. Make sure that you talk about it and make a new plan instead of just abandoning the whole process.

Step 10: Evaluate your progress after a reasonable period (usually five to seven days).

Your evaluation of the progress you've made must be based on input from both you and the woman. If only one of you is feeling better, the other is probably sacrificing too much. Make sure your compromise has struck the right balance.

The planning of Deb and Carlos' trip went smoothly. They were able to agree on all of the preparations, including the budget. Because of the expense, they chose to drive. The trip was tiring but not too uncomfortable. Deb accidentally left her make-up bag at home, but Carlos got big points for telling her he wouldn't want her to be made up anyway! They didn't talk about breast cancer the whole time. During their vacation, Deb at first deliberately stayed away from the subject of breast cancer and her feelings of depression because she knew they were trying to limit those discussions. Carlos, in turn, felt that she was holding back. On the second night, they finally had a long talk about it. Carlos felt that it was repetitive of previous conversations, but he was patient. Over the remaining days of their vacation they had sex twice and talked about cancer three times. They were glad they hadn't scheduled anything, because Deb often didn't even want to get out of bed until the afternoon. Carlos got a little bored, but they both felt less stressed and got lots of sleep.

When they got back, Deb chose her mother, her sister, and a close girlfriend as her three new supports. Talking to these women was great for her because they provided a female perspective that Deb had missed when most of her talks were with Carlos. Deb's sister and friend were often busy, although they tried their best to make time for her, but Deb's mother was always available. Carlos felt a little jealous of the "girls' club," as he thought of it. He wished his own support had been enough, but he never mentioned it until he and Deb did their COPE Step 10 evaluation. Deb then told him that he had nothing to worry about—he was still the most important and most helpful person in her life. After that, Carlos confessed that he was relieved she had more people to give her advice and support and was feeling less burdened.

As you can see, the results for Deb and Carlos were mixed, although generally positive. It's rare that a plan will work out perfectly, so sometimes "pretty good" is actually very good. Hopefully you and the woman you love have made real progress.

There are lots of reasons why a plan might not succeed. If yours hasn't, ask yourself why. Maybe your plan never had a chance because of simple logistics. Maybe your job interferes with dancing lessons, or Deb finds out that her painting doesn't express anything except runny portraits of the cat. So what? Sometimes things don't work out, but that doesn't mean you aren't committed. Try something new.

On the other hand, maybe your plan didn't work for a more serious reason. Perhaps you didn't try hard enough to stick to your plan. If you suspect this is true, question your commitment and the woman's commitment to resolving this particular problem. If one of you has been feeling bitter or unwilling all along, try the problem from a different angle, or try a different problem altogether. It is also possible that the solution you chose was ineffective. Maybe it just didn't affect the problem the way you hoped it would. If this seems like the case, go back to your list of brainstormed suggestions. Try listing some more pros and cons.

If your plan has backfired, all you can do is admit it and try again. This is hard stuff. Just remind each other that you're committed to making things work, no matter what it takes. Setbacks should be expected. As long as you are still trying, you haven't failed.

If the situation has significantly improved, continue with your plan. If the problem is already gone, congratulations!

If you don't feel you've made progress, you should look back over the COPE Model steps and rethink your choices. Does the problem you identified really get at the heart of the situation? Is your goal reasonable? If so, you should try a different solution from the creative list you brainstormed.

Caregiving for Men: A Practical Guide

This isn't an easy time to be a man. What is expected of us has changed a lot in recent years. Men are still supposed to be strong, independent, reliable providers, which can be quite a challenge in itself. But these days men are asked to be emotionally available as well. The two demands probably seem somewhat contradictory, and to be honest, they can be. When we ask women what they really want from us, they're likely to say, "It depends."

Male characteristics like physical strength and aggressiveness have become less valuable with society's increasing dependence on trained professionals operating computers and machines. Communication, cooperation, and sensitivity are now what is needed to function successfully in a working environment. This means that men need to reevaluate the skills they bring to the table.

The double-bind of expectations on men can also put significant strain on male-female relationships. Have you ever seen a guy on the phone with his girlfriend, reluctant to say "I love you" because his buddies are around? Although he's probably making his girlfriend angry, he's not doing it because he's a bad person. He's just caught between his own expectations of what a man should act like, and *hers*. Women don't typically have as much trouble putting their feelings into words because of the expectation that they are "supposed" to express emotion, and because their brains are wired differently. In fact, much of what makes you a man is hard-wired in your brain, so some of the behavior that is expected of you may not be realistic at all. Understanding how to maximize your true potential can help you find new ways to be proud of being a man. Despite the biological distinction between the sexes, however, it remains clear that both women and men have the ability to solve problems, communicate, and work cooperatively.

So now the woman you love has breast cancer, and suddenly you are her caregiver. Maybe you've taken on this role before for a sick relative or friend, but many men have never been called on to help someone back to health, especially over an extended period of time. It's just not something men are commonly asked to do. Men in your position are usually very willing to help, but they often lack the skills. Wanting to be strong, they also forget to take care of themselves, which makes it near-impossible to take care of the woman.

This section will help you learn about the practical

demands of caring for a woman with breast cancer, and yourself, too. Although no one ever wants to have to deal with it, many people find that illness creates an opportunity for women and men to support each other and achieve a closeness they never knew was possible. If you are willing to learn and are open to a new interpretation of what it means to be a strong man, your relationship with the woman you love can not only survive, but thrive.

Taking Care of Her

As a primary member of the woman's committed "team," you need to be directly involved in her care. Even if you've had some experience in caring for sick people, women with breast cancer have some very specific needs, and you will have to learn how to meet them.

Although you and others will be taking charge of her care, make sure the woman is always aware of what is going on. Keeping information back or trying to protect her by sheltering her almost always creates unnecessary tension and fear. Families do best when they act as a coordinated unit and when everyone understands the mission at hand. Open communication will also allow her to tell you about any changes that arise in her needs.

Make her life easier

Until now, the woman has been responsible for a significant share of the household duties that keep your family and/or relationship running smoothly. Now, as you have probably already realized, her contribution will be limited. It's up to you to pick up the slack.

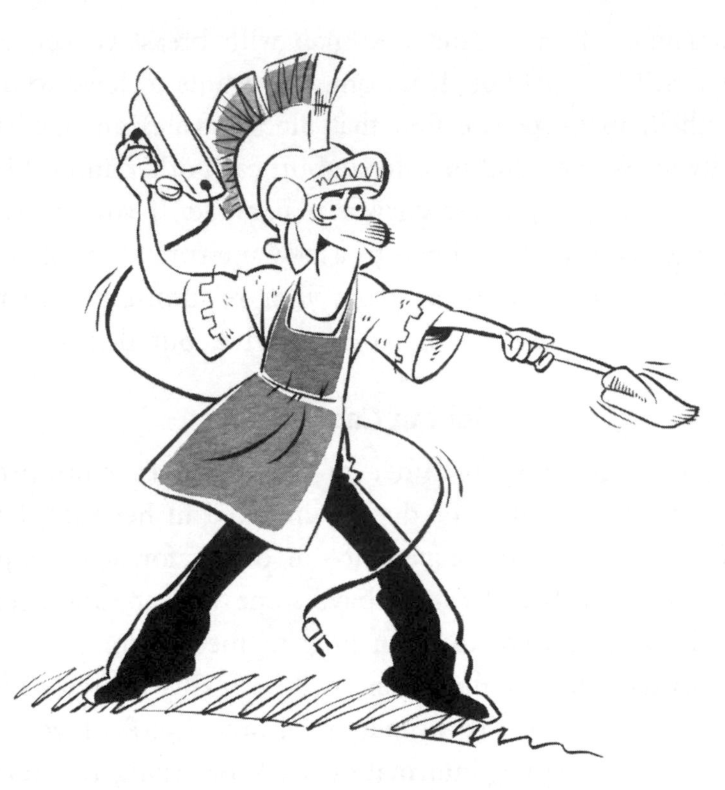

Cooking and cleaning are chores that are often relegated to women. Even if you've never made pasta or scrubbed a toilet, don't feel like you have to invest in a maid service (although if it fits into your budget, it might not be a bad idea). Ask for help and advice from others.

You can also run interference between the woman and any friends, family, or acquaintances who may become overbearing or whom she does not want to see. Don't be hesitant to tell even close relatives and friends that she's not feeling up to a social visit. You have the right to protect her by making her excuses. (But be sure to ask her what she wants first—don't guess at her feelings.)

These are some simple things you can do to make her life a little easier:

- Make her favorite meal
- Do the laundry
- Take care of children
- Screen telephone calls
- Give updates to friends and family
- Keep her gas tank filled
- Share the remote.
- Talk to the doctor, nurse, and social worker
- If you can't attend a doctor's appointment, make sure someone else does
- Plan small vacations
- Manage the medical bills
- Pick up medications
- Schedule counseling sessions
- Help her avoid unfulfilling social engagements
- Allow her control over her environment

Help fill her time with meaningful activity

Setting aside time to talk is essential, but the woman might also enjoy planned activities that you can do together. Her lifestyle will change to adapt to her illness, and this could leave her with a lot of free time. Help her fill it with fun, rewarding projects that could take her mind off her illness.

Here are a few things you can do together, or that you can encourage her to try independently:

- Take up a new hobby
- Shop

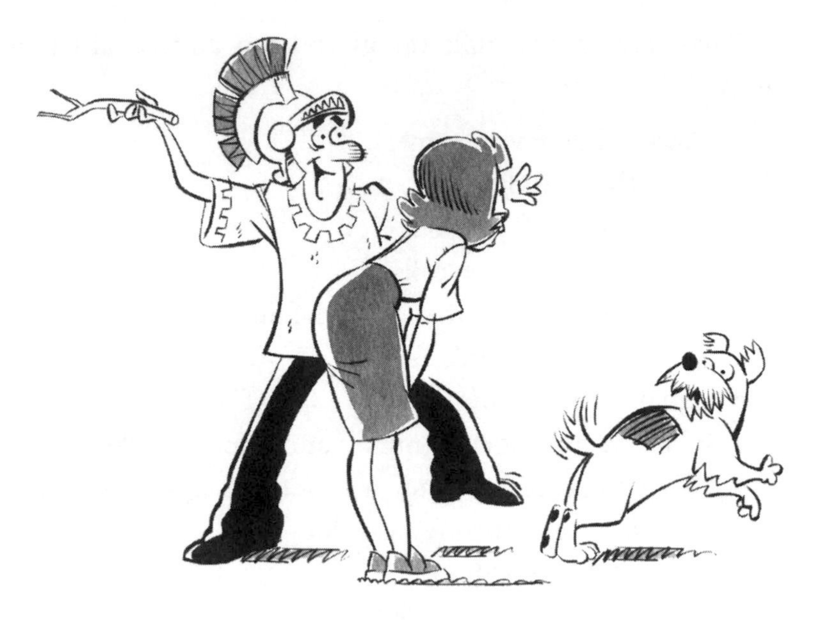

- Exercise
- Cook new recipes
- Dance
- Attend concerts or plays
- Write letters
- Write stories
- Keep a journal or blog
- Watch old movies
- Learn to play an instrument
- Build a website
- Play with a family pet
- Volunteer
- Become politically active
- Go to church
- Join a club

- Read
- Interact with her colleagues from work

Working with the health care team

The best source for accurate information about your loved one's illness, treatment, and recovery is the health care team:

From the physician, you will receive information about the diagnosis, the best course of treatment, the most common side effects of recommended treatment, and the prognosis (most probable outcome).

From the nurse, you will be able to learn how to manage side effects, understand the meaning of the tests, and anticipate common physical problems. Nurses are often the most accessible members of the health care team and can be incredibly helpful in supporting your efforts to understand the complex information and decisions you may have to make.

From the social worker, you should receive emotional support as well as problem solving assistance for you and your family. The social worker should be an advocate for you in the hospital system and the community.

Each team member has a different expertise, but a good team will frequently overlap in the services they provide. As the man, you may frequently be called upon to talk with specific members of the team about a concern or problem. The team should always be the first stop for accurate information. Although the internet, articles, talk-shows, and all too often well-meaning family and friends will make suggestions, these are second-rate sources, as only your health care team truly knows the specific facts of the situation. In fact, you may have to ask family and friends to stop offering medical advice, as this can create fear and confusion in the woman with cancer and in you.

You can say to them, "I know how much you care and that you're trying to help. But you don't know the specifics of the situation. It also makes us feel like you are criticizing us. So if you really want to help us, please do not offer medical advice. But please *do* offer us your time, a small gift, or just a heartfelt word."

Taking Care Of Yourself

Evidence shows that men tend to ignore their own physical and psychological needs much more than women do. It has even been suggested that one of the reasons women live an average of seven years longer than men is because of men's tendency to believe they are indestructible. For too many men, admitting that they are indeed vulnerable means admitting weakness. In reality, refusing to admit that you are human is the true weakness, and dangerous as well. Preventable tragedies occur when people ignore important bodily signals.

When a loved one has an illness, it is common for family members to sacrifice their own needs in an attempt to help. Remember, if you become ill yourself you won't be able to help anyone. Taking good care of yourself is the best way to make sure you'll always be available to the woman you love. So rather than giving up what makes you happy, you may have to cut back doing the things you enjoy. Given the realities of the situations, these activities can help you to be a better caregiver by taking care of yourself. Guilt

Danger Signs	Call the Physician	Call a Mental Health Professional
Thoughts of suicide	X	X
Refusal of treatment without adequate discussion	X	X
Anxiety	X	X
Depression	X	X
Intense, sustained anger	X	X
Violent behavior	X	X
Social withdrawal	X	X
Confusion	X	
Physical pain	X	
Not eating and drinking	X	
Sleep extremes (insomnia or sleeping all the time)	X	
Incontinence	X	
Unable/unwilling to talk	X	X
Prolonged, uncontrollable crying	X	X

should never get in the way of having a realistic approach to what you can actually do for her and what you need to stay healthy for yourself. (For more ideas, see the COPE exercise on page 62.)

Don't (always) grin and bear it.

Men often see it as their job to be brave and optimistic to keep the woman's spirits up, which is great. But they forget to take into account the emotional impact that breast cancer is having on them. It's impossible to hide strained feelings from others for any long period of time, especially from someone who knows you as well as this woman does. Nobody is that good of an actor. Pretending to be cheerful and refusing to acknowledge stress will only add to her concerns. She'll worry that you're going to crack under the pressure—and she'll be right to worry.

Don't try to escape your feelings.

Withdrawing is probably the worst thing you can do to yourself and to the woman you love. Putting off questions about your feelings, focusing solely on her physical needs to avoid talk of emotions, drinking, and drug abuse are all ways of withdrawing. You may think you are maintaining a manly stoicism, but she'll probably just think you are too fragile to handle an open discussion. Running away from whatever's bothering you makes you seem weak and demonstrates that you can't face reality.

Look after your physical health.

Preoccupied as you are, it will be all too easy to let go of your ordinary daily health routine. The big problems in your life can quickly overwhelm the little stuff. Men tend to underestimate the heavy toll that physical deficiencies (of nutrition, exercise, sleep, etc.) take on their ability to bear up under pressure. So shave, eat a balanced meal, get some rest, et cetera—even if you have to force yourself. If it helps, make a list of things to do in the morning and before bed. It might seem ridiculous, but with your mind on breast cancer, you probably won't be thinking about brushing your teeth.

Tell her about your concerns.

It goes without saying that right now, she is more vulnerable than you are. You are already prepared to make allowances for her illness, which is important and necessary. Breast cancer *will* change the dynamic of your interaction, but it shouldn't alter it completely. A relationship between a man and a woman is a partnership, and no matter what the circumstances, partnerships are built on mutual support.

Of course you don't want to burden a sick woman with your problems. That's understandable. But think of the situation from her perspective. Hiding your own hurt cuts off her access to you. Breast cancer shouldn't force her to be less of a wife or lover—she needs constants in her life now more than ever. Talking about your feelings and concerns might even take her mind off her own troubles for a while. The key is waiting until the time is right.

Seeking Social Support

Who can help?

Because men often do not reach out to others when

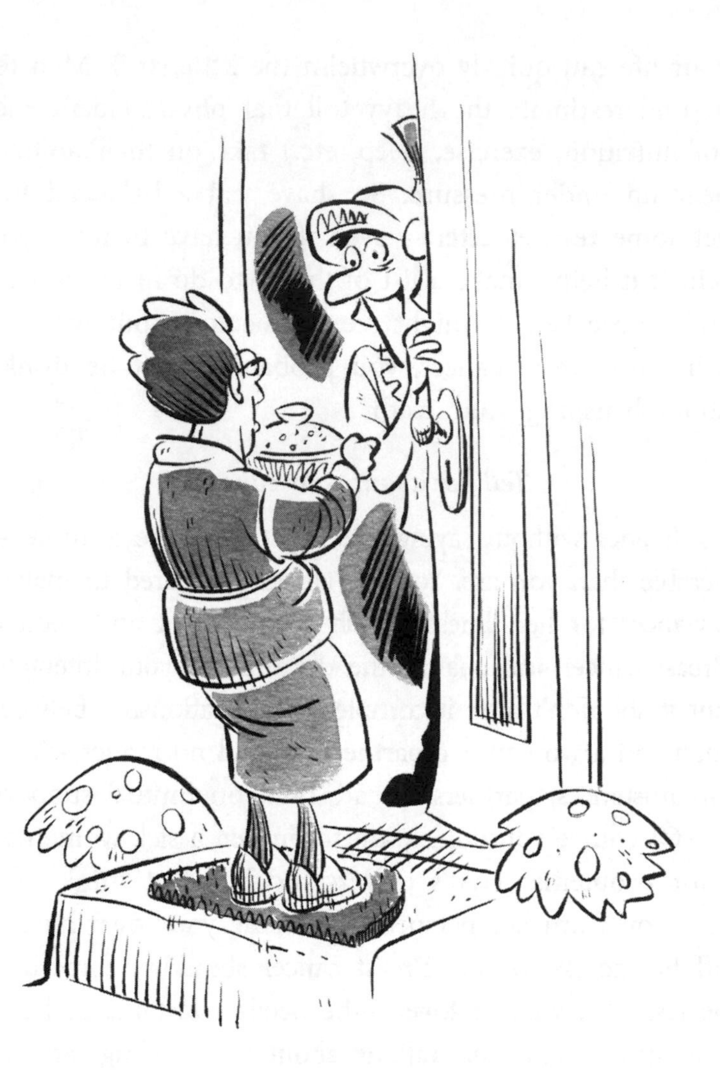

they have personal problems, it is hard for them to understand how comforting the woman may find the support of her community. Men are often astonished how people seem to come out of the woodwork to help out. But guys, you *do* have to come out of your comfort zone and ask.

Other men and women who have had similar experiences may approach you and offer help. Do not say no. Talk to them about how they coped. What resources did they find helpful? What wasn't worth the effort? Also, by attending a support group you will quickly become knowledgeable about available resources.

Some of the most common places to find social support are places of worship, community centers, mental health centers, cancer related support groups like the Wellness Community, the American Cancer Society, your local community hospital (especially the social work department), unions, and social clubs. Of course, an Internet search will also provide a wealth of additional information.

You will be quite surprised by how many people are out there and are just waiting to be asked for assistance. But remember, you need to take the first step, as many people who are willing to help may also be concerned about your privacy and hesitant to approach you directly.

How can they help?

The kind of help you need will determine where you should look for assistance. Money is a problem for many people confronted with cancer. If it is in your case, look into your eligibility for government programs first; Medicaid, Medicare, and Social Security Disability should be your first stops. Do not skip this step. Next, look into state-run programs for people affected by serious illness. You can call your congressional representative's office to find out about organizations and other resources in your community. If you belong to a place of worship, you should also let them know about any problems you have.

The Knights of Columbus, Masons, Elks, and Moose Lodges may have programs for people in need in your community. Although local community groups seldom help out financially, they will provide food, car rides, and respite for caregivers and will help advocate for other assistance. There are many small community based social support groups, especially for breast cancer (be sure to check the Resources listed at the back of this book) who will know best what is available in your area. For example, if you need medications that you cannot afford, most pharmaceutical companies do have free drug programs. But again, you must apply.

The world is filled with good people who want to help, but you must reach out to them first. Although this might not come naturally to you, it is the wise and courageous thing to do.

Health Insurance and Advocacy

Anyone who has confronted cancer knows that there is a major health insurance crisis in the United States. There are about 47 million people with no health insurance at all, and many more than that with inadequate health insurance. Recent national studies have demonstrated that approximately fifty percent of personal bankruptcies in the United States are from some form of medical debt.

Unfortunately, most cancer care is now determined not

by a patient's needs, but by his or her insurance policy. Cost, rather than quality, is now what determines medical care. Insurance co-pays and deductibles have a devastating impact on people with cancer and their families.

This comes at a time when hospitals are closing and are overwhelmed by the costs of the uninsured or under-insured. More employers are refusing to provide basic health care coverage to most of their employees. Some incredibly profitable companies continue to put pressure on other companies to further reduce health insurance benefits. This race to the bottom is expected to put working women who are too young for Medicare at great risk because women are much less likely than men to be provided with health insurance by their employer.

Health insurance companies are businesses that must make a profit. Nevertheless, it is possible to personalize your interactions. If there is a problem with your health insurance, start with the person who is assigned to you and try to speak to that same person each time. Always be honest and civil; if you receive an answer you don't think is acceptable, ask to speak with the supervisor. Keep notes on all of your conversations, and be persistent! Make the company realize you will never give up.

You might have to be quite forceful in advocating for the woman with breast cancer. You can't trust the health insurance company, or, in too many cases, the physicians who work for them, to be totally objective. Always demand a second opinion and even a third if necessary. Never passively accept a decision that comes at the detriment of the woman you love.

Applying the Cope Model

When people fail to pay attention to their own basic needs, they begin to feel frustrated and angry. This is normal, but avoidable. Guys, it doesn't have to be this way. When people are under stress they tend to see things in terms of black and white and right and wrong, with nothing in between. This way of managing problems wastes energy and is usually unrealistic. In a hurricane the unbending tree always falls first; life is about being and being flexible when necessary. The choice to be flexible is under your direct control. Fortunately, the COPE Model is all about endless possibilities and options.

So, let's use COPE now to mange a very common and complex problem that men confront when supporting woman while she is still in active treatment.

The Problem

How do I meet my own needs while not feeling guilty about not being there every second to support the woman I love?

Remember—a problem is something that you can influence or manage better *and* that you care enough about to invest energy in very soon, like today or tomorrow.

Expert Information

Being brutally honest with yourself, as a man, what do you find engaging, relaxing, distracting, meaningful, pleasurable, fun? What has given you pleasure in the past? Make a very short list of the ways you feel most rejuvenated and refreshed.

Creativity and Optimism

Now brainstorm things you can do that will be pleasurable for you. Remember, that brainstorming is a time when you must suspend any judgments about the options you create. Just write them all down. Reality is not a part of this process.

> Brainstorming: Golf once a week, take cooking classes, spend more time with grandchildren, go on short vacation with family, take art classes, go to gym, get a personal trainer, go to movies, read a book, write a book, have drinks with friends at least once every two weeks, walk at least thirty minutes every day, call a friend from college, get a medical check-up, read a book to her, go away with a good friend for one weekend every month, buy a new car, sell the new expensive boat, take longer showers, get new reading glasses, get a message, make a list of things that need to be fixed around the house and get someone else to fix them, plant flowers, learn to play the harmonica, buy new tools you don't need, build something with your hands, buy new clothes, buy something for the woman in your life, write her a poem, help your children to write about this experience, write a list of the sad and good things that have come from this experience, ask the woman what you two can do together that would make you both feel good about yourselves, volunteer your time at a local charity, get a dog or some other pet, go to great restaurant on your own or with a friend, talk to a counselor.

Okay, okay, I came up with all of these. Why don't you add at least five more?

Planning

Now just take a few of the options above and judge (with brutal honesty) which you are you most likely to do in the very near future. Which will take the least amount of effort and give you the greatest amount of pleasure or meaning with the least amount of guilt?

We have found that when men do this exercise with the woman in their life and other family members, they find it fun and find great relief in knowing they have the wisdom and courage to work *together.* It also makes the woman feel more connected at a time when isolation is all too common. For men, having this role-modeling ability sends a very powerful message to their family: whatever happens, we will support each other and protect our individuality.

Coping with the Phases of Breast Cancer

A woman with breast cancer always needs physical care, expert medical information, and emotional support. But as her body progresses through the stages of her illness, the specifics of those needs will change. This chapter provides a roadmap to the phases of breast cancer so you will know what to expect, when to expect it, and how to adjust your behavior accordingly. Keep in mind, however, that skills relating to communication, problem solving, and caregiving will be useful during *every* stage of breast cancer.

Also remember that not every woman will experience the phases of breast cancer the same way. Doctors know a lot about breast cancer, so it *is* possible to predict the most common reactions to diagnosis, treatment, and so on. Still, no woman should be treated as a "breast cancer patient" in the impersonal sense. She is a unique individual and the only one who knows for sure how she feels. If you are able to communicate effectively, you will be able to identify her needs based on her input as well as the information that follows.

Men are often at a loss as to what they can provide when the assistance is not tangible (money, food, gifts, et cetera). When it comes to emotional and spiritual needs, we tend to struggle. Women do not want quick fixes or answers from men. Women want a meaningful connection. In many ways, this is what they want from us under most circumstances.

Remember that what is meaningful to women may not be obvious to us men. Women value physical presence and verbal communication. Just acting in a loving manner may not be enough; you may have to put your feelings into words. Tell her that you will be there no matter what happens.

For many people, caring for someone at the end of life is an extremely rewarding experience. Most people who choose to avoid being near dying loved ones later regret their decision. No one can guarantee what your experience will be like, but you might never again have the opportunity to connect with someone who needs you so badly.

During each phase of breast cancer, the woman will have three primary needs. She needs to take *Action*, or to have action taken on her behalf. She needs to have her questions answered—that is, *Knowledge*. Finally, she needs emotional *Support* from you and others.

Diagnosis of Breast Cancer

When a woman learns she has breast cancer, disbelief or even stunned confusion are normal and to be expected. The news is extremely upsetting and difficult to understand. Once she is able to process it, typically her first objective is to learn more about the disease and find the best place to get medical treatment. At the same time, she is also concerned about how her illness and treatment will affect her loved ones, including you.

Although at first the shock might feel overwhelming, for her sake you must get a grip on your own feelings.

Generally, just after the diagnosis the woman will receive an outpouring of attention from family and friends. While their support and compassion can be helpful and comforting, it can also be overwhelming. (For tips on how to handle an outpouring of outside help, check out "Seeking Social Support" on page 57 in the "Caregiving for Men" chapter.)

Some family members and friends, on the other hand, may be so deeply shaken by the diagnosis that they withdraw entirely. They may avoid the woman and even you, leaving both of you hurt and confused. If this happens, recognize that these people are reacting not to you or the woman personally, but to a situation that makes them very uncomfortable. Their inability to cope with others' illnesses is their own problem, and while you may understandably be sad that they can't overcome their feelings for the woman's sake, try not to be angry. You can play a useful role by seeking them out and talking over the situation. If you approach them on friendly and understanding terms, you may be able to persuade them to re-engage with the woman at a time when she needs them most.

Past experiences with unhappy and stressful events will give you clues as to how the woman might try to cope with the diagnosis of breast cancer. In fact, the diagnosis and the struggle to decide the best form of treatment could bring back feelings of fear and vulnerability from other very difficult times. However, what has worked in the past might not work now. This is likely to be the most difficult and intense struggle of her life. Luckily, she has you to help her through it.

Taking Action

Since men usually value actions over words, this is when we really rise to the occasion. But that doesn't mean you need to take on everything by yourself—far from it. Women who play an active role in the decision-making process concerning their medical care almost always make a better psychological adjustment over time. However, this is a generalization, so you should try to find out how active she wants to be in the decision-making process.

The woman needs to identify a medical surgical or radiation oncologist whom she trusts and has confidence in. You can help by asking the primary care physician for a referral, talking to your friends, and getting a second opinion. She also needs to gain access to information and consultations to help understand the complex medical information pertaining to her treatment.

Accompany her on medical visits and listen in on phone conversations with doctors (but only if she wants you to).

Take careful notes and ask questions during all medical consultations. Unless you're going to lose your job, be there! Or get a family member or friend to go with her. No one should have to go to a doctor visit alone when the stakes are so high. It is also helpful to tape-record the visit so you can later reinforce what was said and share the information with other family members. When in doubt, reach out to a licensed mental health professional who specializes in caring for cancer patients and their loved ones.

Gaining Knowledge

After the shock of a breast cancer diagnosis, a whole host of questions suddenly arises. Here are some common concerns:

- Am I going to die?

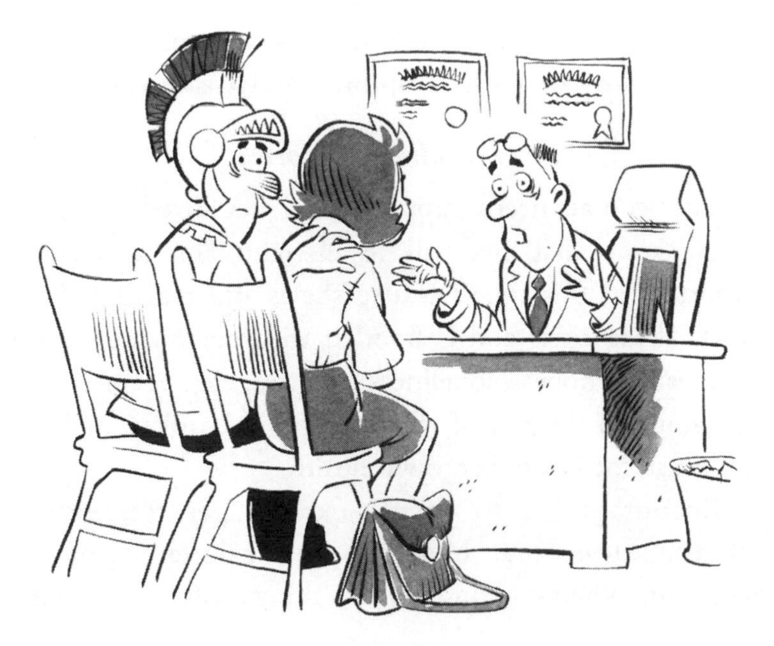

- Will the cancer be controlled? Has the cancer spread beyond the breast?
- How much will all of this cost? Will I go broke?
- Am I getting the proper medical care?
- Will there be unpleasant physical changes?
- Can I still function and be productive?
- Will I be able to return to work?
- How will this impact my loved ones?
- Will I be too much of a burden?
- How will I manage feelings of guilt?
- Will I be abandoned?
- What about my children? Is this genetic?
- Who will take care of my loved ones while I am sick or if I die?

You can help at this early stage by researching where she can receive the best care and attention and by learning as much as possible about breast cancer. Familiarize yourself with common symptoms and treatments.

Providing Support

The woman needs support from her loved ones, and also to know that they will be all right. This is especially important at this time because she is still reacting to the shock of the crisis and is flooded with her own emotions (like fear, numbness, loneliness, sadness, etc). Let her know that you and the rest of the family will be okay, and that she must focus on her own health.

Encourage her to openly express her concerns by listening, touching, hugging, and asking supportive questions. When you do this, two things will happen. First, your relationship will deepen and the woman will be better able to control her fears about the illness and its treatment. Second, you will be called upon to discuss some difficult issues. You will need to listen sympathetically while she talks about her possible death, even if it is not a likely possibility. This takes courage. However, now is the time to establish that she can talk to you about *anything.* This opportunity may not come again.

Don't say that everything will be all right, because you don't know for sure. But do try to stay positive. Tell her you will be there for her no matter what. Also, talk to family and close friends to be sure they are aware of what is happening and know how to show they care.

During Treatment

Psychological distress is usually at its highest when the treatment begins, after which it slowly decreases over time.

Since breast cancer is frequently cured, the outlook for most newly-diagnosed women with localized cancer to the breast only is very good. If the cancer has already spread, the goal of treatment is to control the disease, because acheiving a cure is no longer a reality.

If the woman is even remotely interested in having children in the future, it is important that she consult a fertility expert before treatment begins. You should not assume that you know how she will feel about potentially losing her ability to bear children. Ask her directly.

Treatment may carry any number of side effects. But the good news is that most of these are temporary, and eventually her original quality of life will return.

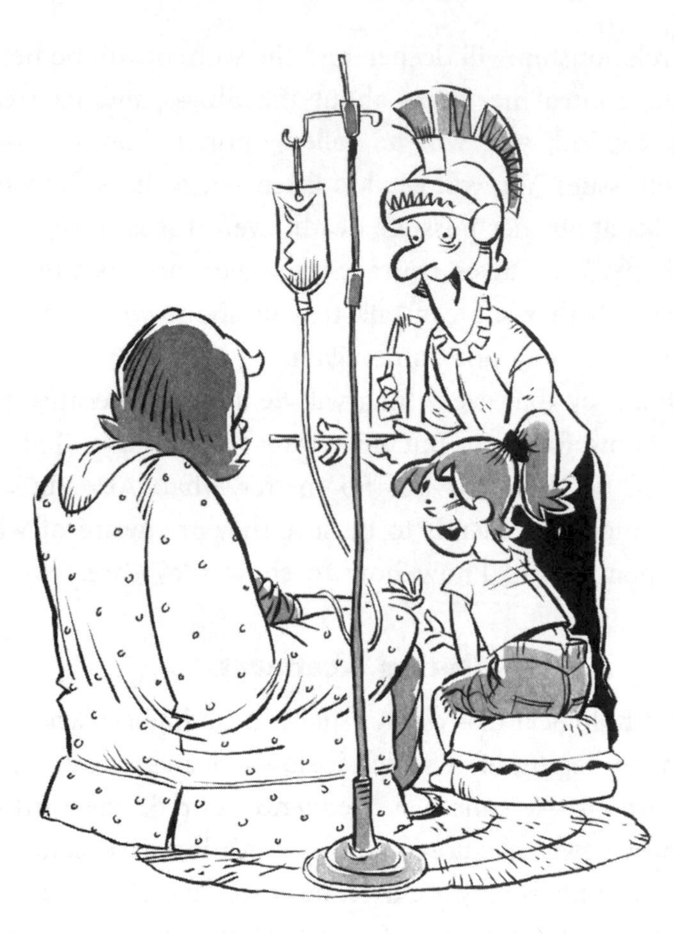

Taking Action

Talk to the doctor to learn about treatment. Make sure to ask about symptom management (control of pain, nausea, fatigue, et cetera). This way, both of you will understand what's going on and be confident that she is receiving the best treatment available.

Accompany the woman to key medical appointments in which decisions about the treatment are being made.

Volunteer to do this so she doesn't feel she has to ask. If you can't be at all the appointments or treatments, arrange for someone else to accompany her. Most people simply are not able to hear and understand medical informaiton due to the stress of the physician visit. Two sets of ears are always better than one.

If, after treatment, the woman continues to experience unpleasant symptoms such as anxiety, weight gain, and fatigue, consult the physician.

Gaining Knowledge

These are some of the questions she might ask:

- Is the treatment likely to cure or at least control the cancer?
- How will it impact my family?
- How long will the treatment take?
- What physical changes will I experience?

The woman needs to know that the physician and treatment she has chosen are best suited to her needs and will ensure the best chance for a cure. Her physician should be able to provide her with information and resources relating to image recovery.*

Providing Support

Again: talk to her. Remind her that the process is expected to be demanding, and that's not her fault. Ask

**Image recovery* means maximizing attractiveness with wigs, make-up, and accessories to lessen or hide any unpleasant physical changes.

her how she is managing on a regular basis; her feelings are probably in constant flux.

Remember, if you are really serious about doing your best to help the woman cope with breast cancer, your physical presence, honest communication, and support are always the most helpful strategies.

The great news is that women say it means a lot to them when they have a supportive man in their lives during treatment. Even if you can't be there each and every day, in the long run, your perseverance will make a big difference.

Remission or Cure

Although the woman will definitely be glad to have finally finished treatment, she may also feel vulnerable or even threatened. This fear usually stems from her awareness that nothing is being done anymore to control the cancer. This can be very scary. We all find solace in *doing something* to fight against what's wrong.

Once the woman relaxes and releases the energy she focused on treatment, she is often left with a sense of emptiness. Re-entry into daily living can feel very mundane, and she may spend time re-evaluating the things she once valued. On the other hand, she may also feel relieved, or even that her life has new meaning. These two reactions might sound contradictory, but the same woman can experience both, even at the same time.

The transition from active treatment to observation can also disrupt her family. Emotions can run very high as everyone comes to fully realize the toll the illness has taken.

Taking Action

Just because treatment is over doesn't mean there's nothing left to be done. Actually, for most women the end of treatment can be a very unsettling time. But this is a time when you can really help. As the man, you should have a clear understanding of what your loved one has to do to try to stay healthy. Show your caring and demonstrate your committment by getting involved in a respectful, healthy way. Encouraging her to take medications on time, follow through on doctors' appointments, eat healthy, and get plenty of rest is a convincing way to show love and concern. It is especially important that you actively support the woman in taking prescribed medications. Once she is off hospital-based treatment, there is likely to be a dramatic decrease in compliance with medical regimens. This is a very serious problem. Using COPE together to keep her on track can bring you closer together and enable the woman to regain her sense of independence and self control.

Keep in mind that the time when active hospital-based treatment ends is always a time of reflection and of managing fears of recurrence. Contact with the health care team will be dramatically reduced, which could lead to fears due to lower levels of surveillance. After months of careful medical monitoring, the woman might find herself frightened by this anticipated and welcome milestone, and she is likely to worry that cancer will recur.

You can stay actively involved in the woman's care by attending follow-up medical visits, keeping track of future appointments, and asking questions about the surveillance plan. But most of all, this is a time when the woman will need to reflect on her experience with you and others. Your lives will hopefully begin to settle into a more comfortable, "normal" routine. You're shifting down from "crisis gear," so taking definitive action is now less important than providing emotional support on a daily basis.

Gaining Knowledge

The woman should be monitored by her physician for any changes in her medical status.

These are some questions she might have during remission/after being cured:

- How will I know if the cancer recurs? What should I be looking out for?
- What will we do if it does recur?
- How do other women cope with the fear of recurrence?
- When is it safe for me to become pregnant?
- What changes can I expect in my sexual functioning as a result of this treatment?
- How long till I can resume a normal sex life?
- How can I manage problems such as vaginal drying or decreased sex drive?

Providing Support

Even though almost all women who are diagnosed with localized early stage breast cancer will be cured, no one can guarantee that it will not return. Be honest about your concerns, realistic or not, and encourage her to express hers.

She might be worried that the cancer will recur, that your relationship won't be the same again, or even that she'll die. Don't dismiss these fears, even if you only mean to reassure her. Treat every concern seriously, but let her know that you're hopeful and willing to work on whatever the future brings.

Only give advice if she asks for it first and, if she does, make sure she knows that she does not have to follow your advice. Remember, when in doubt, reach out to a licensed mental health professional with expertise in caring for cancer patients and their loved ones.

Two or three months after the treatment ends, children and other loved ones might begin talking about the experience. You can help them open up by starting the conversation. Tell them your thoughts and concerns about the crisis.

Recurrence of Cancer

Although most women will be cured of their breast cancer, for some cancer will return. Cancer recurs because of the limitations of treatment, *not* because of anything the woman did or did not do.

For most women, the discovery of a recurrence will be much more distressing than the original diagnosis, even though it might be less shocking. This may be because they are aware that the prognosis is not as positive for recurrence as it is for localized breast cancer. Sometimes, the woman is worn down by the demands of the illness and its treatment.

Other women may feel that because they have already

been through the diagnosis and know what to expect, they have acquired new coping skills and have a stable support system. These women may find the recurrence less stressful than the original diagnosis. Either way, you should understand that no woman wants to be told that she has a recurrence of breast cancer since the focus of treatment then shifts to controlling the disease rather than curing it.

As always, it is the man's responsibility to be physically available, communicative, honest, supportive, and hopeful.

Taking Action

One of your responsibilities is to start the conversation about how the family will make adjustments to support the woman while still functioning properly. Make sure that she is always an active participant in these conversations so she doesn't feel even more isolated and/or burdensome.

Remember, if either of you have any specific financial concerns or worries, you must talk about them openly and work together to overcome them. Financial resources are frequently an important concern during recurrence.

Attend as many of her meetings with the physician as you can, just as you did when treatment first began.

Gaining Knowledge

Encourage a meeting with the oncologist as soon as possible to discuss treatment options and explore such concerns as:

- What are the costs and benefits of treatment?
- Will it be paid for by her insurance?

- What is her prognosis?
- What will happen if there is a shift to palliative care* only?

Providing Support

The woman needs two kinds of support. First, she needs the certainty that she will not be abandoned by her health care team or her family. Second, she needs people she can count on to be there for her and to be her advocate.

This can be a terrifying time for the woman and her family. She should be surrounded by people who are kind, patient, and accepting of her response to recurrence, whatever it may be.

You may need to protect her from people who insist that something she did caused the cancer to return. This is not the time for the woman to be feeling any unnecessary guilt or shame.

Express your own disappointment and fear, but be sure to be very sympathetic and reassure her that the situation is nobody's fault. Make it clear that the two of you will work together to get her the best possible care.

End of Life

Most women who are diagnosed during the early stages of breast cancer will not die from the illness. Because breast cancer is usually cured, it is especially sad when a woman's life is significantly shortened by it.

The role of the man in this situation—whether as a

**Palliative care* combines the active treatment of physical symptoms by a physician and nurse with the psychosocial aspects of care for the patient and family by a social worker. It focuses on care over cure.

husband, son, father, in-law, or close friend—is very important. The road to the end of the woman's life is filled with difficult emotions and challenges. If the dying process is prolonged, it will be especially stressful for the woman and the family. However, her need for close emotional connections to you and other important people is likely to increase.

Taking Action

Accompany her to the physician's appointment to be certain that everything possible has, in fact, been done. Your presence at the physician visit will alert the health care team of your role and the need to keep you informed and involved in decision making. It will also make the woman feel much safer.

Meet with the woman and everyone concerned to openly discuss the situation. (You should first ask the woman if she will feel comfortable in this setting.) First, everyone present should clearly commit to being there for her. Then you should open up a discussion of any possible worries, real or imagined. Carefully explore whether or not there are any other options, such as clinical trials.* Be sure not to pressure the woman—she'll talk if she wants to, and hopefully she'll speak up if she isn't happy with what you're doing.

This is an especially important time to remember to keep the children informed and supported. Please see page 100 for information on Children and Breast Cancer.

---

*A *clinical trial* tests the effectiveness of the newest promising treatments, or might be focused on making new discoveries to help patients.

Invite the palliative care team to be part of a family meeting so they can advise the family on how you can all work together to make this time easier. You can help maximize the quality of life during her final days by learning about symptom management. Any creditable palliative care team will grant you immediate access to a physician, nurse, social worker, and chaplain. If these elements are not readily available, quickly find a new team to work with.

If (and only if) the woman is interested, this is also the time to discuss and plan burial or crematory arrangements. Find out if she wants anything in particular read at her funeral or engraved on her tombstone. She may be uncomfortable thinking about these things, so be delicate.

Gaining Knowledge

The woman needs to be absolutely positive that nothing more can be done to control her breast cancer. She also needs to know that everything will be done to maximize the quality of her life.

At this point, she may also want to know:

- Will I be abandoned if my death is prolonged?
- Will I be remembered when I am gone?
- Will I still received high-quality care now that there is no longer a chance for recovery?
- How can I create a legacy for my children?

The palliative care team will be able to walk you through the dying process, provide expert symptom management and emotional support for the woman and the family. They should also provide bereavement counseling after her death.

Providing Support

Do not waste time and energy keeping secrets from each other. By now, she should not be afraid to tell you if she is scared, feels worse, or needs something. Continued communication will help her feel that she is still part of the family and has not already been put in the past. Expect intense emotions. Anger, sadness, and crying are not problems; avoidance is a very big problem. Whenever in doubt, reach out to a licensed mental health professional with expertise in caring for cancer patients and their loved ones.

Tell the woman that you will always be available to help her—if this is true. If this is a promise you cannot make, talk openly about making sure that someone else will fulfill that role. For example, if you have your own serious medical health problems you may not be able to be as physically supportive as you would like.

If the period of the end of her life is drawn out, you may begin to feel stuck in a state of constant grief, unable to achieve closure. You might be tempted to pull away from her, emotionally or even physically. This is understandable. You've been under a lot of stress for a long time, and it hurts to see a loved one suffering without hope for recovery. It may feel like the battle is already lost.

But remember, sometimes the quality of the process can be just as important as the result of the mission (see "Mission-Based vs. Process-Based Behavior" on page 10 in the "Communication" chapter). Take full advantage of her remaining time. Though this time will inevitably be sad, it doesn't always have to be tragic. See if she's willing to laugh over the good times you've had. Tell her you love her; make her feel good. Later, you will be proud to remember that you made her final days as happy as possible.

Applying the COPE Model

The Problem

How can I best support this woman at the end of her life?

Remember—a problem is something that you can influence or manage better *and* that you care enough about to invest energy in very soon, like today or tomorrow.

Loving and caring for the dying woman in your life certainly meets this criteria at all levels. We wish you didn't have to be confronted with this reality, as we have experienced this sorrow first-hand. This is hard. We admire your courage in being there for her and your family.

Expert Information

The woman is the best person to tell you what she needs, so you must ask her. *You* are the expert on what you will realistically be able to provide. You must be brutally honest with yourself. Therefore, the expert information you require can only come from an open and honest conversation between you and her. It is also essential that you engage your children, if you have any, in this process. (See the chart on page 100 for tips on talking to children about breast cancer.) By drawing clearly-specified goals from the "sharing process," you can bring out the best in all family members and add meaning to this experience.

This is a great opportunity to share your love, demonstrate your commitment, and show next generation what it means to be wise and courageous.

Creativity and Optimism

Now let's brainstorm some things you can do to *best support this woman at the end of her life.*

Remember that brainstorming is a time when you must suspend any judgments about the options you create. Just write them all down. Reality is not a part of this process. Be open to new ways to best support the woman, as this is your last opportunity to do so.

> Brainstroming: ask her what would be most helpful to her and use that information, ask yourself what you can honestly do with the resources you have, imagine what would she or you would want most if you had unlimited resources , set up daily meetings to talk about what would be supportive today, ask the children how they would like to be supportive, invite family and friends to visit for short periods of time (depending on her energy level), watch old movies together, look at wedding pictures, cry together, make jokes and laugh together, talk seriously, forgive each other, treat your time together like gold, tell her you love her, pray together, have your religious leader come to visit, support and accept her belief systems as they are, touch her, be sure that her symptoms are well managed by the hospice team, advocate for her forcefully if needed, never ever tolerate poor symptom management (especially pain control), write your wills, renew your wedding vows, write letters to the children and grandchildren, make a video, cook her

favorite meals, write her a poem, write her the story of your life together, apologize and let her do the same for past hurts.

Okay, okay, I came up with all of these. Why don't you add at least five more?

Planning

Now just take a few of the options above and judge (with brutal honesty) which you are you most likely to act upon in the very near future. Which will take the least amount of effort, and will give you the greatest satisfaction in knowing that you did what a wise, loving, committed, and courageous man would do to support a person he loves at the end of her life?

When men are there for the women they love in a honest and meaningful way, the sadness and stress they feel tends to fade away over time. But the intense intimacy and personal growth that come with knowing that you were there for your loved one at the end of her life never fade.

Menopause: What Men Can Do

Our society has come a long way toward understanding menopause. We know that it marks the end of fertility, and we know that it is caused by a change in hormone levels that comes naturally with age. "Meano-pause," as some men call it, gets a bad rap for the roller-coaster of physical and emotional changes it brings, but we understand that those changes are normal and to be expected.

Imagine, then, how surprised the supposed experts were to hear that men across the country consider coping with a woman's menopause one of their greatest challenges. In fact, some men who are in your very situation—dealing with cancer in a woman they love—consider the effects of menopause even harder to manage than their fears about her disease.

There's a reason these men (and women with breast cancer) have to worry about menopause more than most people. Cancer treatments can induce the phase in women who are still of childbearing years. Natural menopause may take ten years before estrogen levels in the blood become extremely low and a woman's period completely stops, but a young woman undergoing chemotherapy may go into menopause abruptly and experience more severe effects.

The Facts about Menopause

Believe it or not, menopause occurs naturally in women *and* men. It is triggered by a decrease of hormones—estrogen in women, testosterone in men. Under ordinary circumstances, menopause occurs in women around forty-five to fifty years of age. During that time, her periods may be irregular, occur less frequently, and finally stops permanently.

For men, the hormone decrease can lead to baldness and an unwanted migration of unhygienic-looking hair to the ears and nose. For women, it can lead to hot flashes, mood swings, and a decreased interest in sex. They may also suffer from mood swings and a certain amount of emotional turbulence. (See the opposite page for more details about possible physical and psychological side effects.) No one ever said getting older was easy!

How Cancer Complicates Menopause

About two-thirds of the more than 2 million breast cancer survivors were already experiencing or had already experienced menopause at the time of diagnosis. This is because most women are diagnosed with breast cancer well

Possible Side Effects of Menopause

Psychological	Physical
Feeling old	Hot flashes
Fear	Pain during sexual intercourse
Helplessness	Weakened bladder control
Frustration	Weight gain
Anxiety	Difficulty sleeping
Depression	Fatigue
Shame	Lethargy
Confusion	Night sweats
Isolation	Water retention
Inability to concentrate	Skin irritation
Feeling unattractive and/or undesirable	Headaches
Feeling masculine	Vaginal drying, itching, bleeding, or discharge

after the age of fifty. In fact, the average age of a woman diagnosed with breast cancer is sixty-three. Although movies and soaps tend to portray breast cancer patients as very beautiful, very rich young women who usually die very quickly, most women with breast cancer are older and fortunately will live a long time. Ultimately, most will not die from cancer.

But for the remaining third of breast cancer sufferers, chemotherapy and, to a lesser degree, hormonal therapies might temporarily or permanently cause infertility. A woman who is simultaneously confronted with breast cancer and the strong possibility of not being able to have children after treatment is likely to be highly distressed. *This is why it is so essential for women and men who are being treated for cancer to talk with a counselor about saving eggs or sperm for later use if they would like to have children—BEFORE any treatments begin.* Preserving the possibility of having children can ease some of her (and your) anxiety.

A more troublesome problem may crop up if and when the woman recognizes that her interest in having sex has decreased. She will worry about how this will impact her relationship with you (if you two are married or sexually involved). Should this issue arise, she won't find it helpful if you shy away from an emotional response or dismiss her worries by saying that only saving her life is important. She needs to know that you understand the seriousness of her concerns and will be there for her no matter what happens.

Menopause can be particularly scary when it is brought on by cancer treatments because the onset is so fast. Courageous men will be understanding of the situation and will not allow themselves to become overwhelmed by the highly charged emotional reactions that are likely to result. This is a hard time for both of you, so be honest and muster up your resolve. You will help the woman in your life, and in doing so, you will act like a man you can admire.

Applying the COPE Model

Like many of the issues you will encounter, difficult situations caused by menopause can be greatly improved

DO React By...

Listening

Believing what she tells you

Sharing your own concerns and feelings

Actively participating in problem solving

Being supportive and reassuring

Being respectful of her suffering

Taking on some of the chores

Accepting that role reversals are sometimes inevitable

DON'T React By...

Avoiding the subject

Getting angry in response to her mood swings

Acting like you know what she is going through

Being proud of your ignorance ("I don't want to know!")

Treating her like a child or a helpless patient

Making fun of her

Trying to find an easy fix

Telling her the changes are all in her head

by employing the problem-management skills you learned from the COPE Model. Take this one:

Kevin and Tamara have been married a long time and have had their ups and downs, but it has never been this hard. They feel isolated from one other. Although deeply committed to each other, they are now both frustrated. They talk little and avoid talking in depth about anything. Tamara has no sex drive and Kevin is feeling guilty about wanting to make love with his wife. Kevin explains that because he feels guilty and angry he has avoided touching Tamara. Tamara then feels isolated and abandoned, which she says is her worst fear. Tamara has powerful mood swings where she accuses Kevin of being selfish. Tamara says things that she regrets, and Kevin feels guilty because he does *feel selfish. Kevin and Tamara realize that they have to find new ways of feeling close.*

They both agree that the biggest problem is the Tamara has dramatic mood swings that scare her and that alienate Kevin. Because the mood swings are a big problem for both of them, they are motivated to focus on this first and then sex later. So, they decide to use the COPE model.

Kevin and Tamara define their problem as:

They need a way to respond to moods swings in a way that does not lead to feeling isolated from and frustrated with each other.

After brainstorming a list of solutions without judging one another's ideas, the couple weighs the positives and negatives of a selected handful and decides, after an honest discussion of their feelings, on a few solutions to try over the following three to five days.

The solutions Kevin and Tamara agreed to use were: to talk with a counselor about how to identify sexual activities that are acceptable to both of them, to establish cues to let each other know when they are getting overwhelmed with feelings, and to take a meditation classes together to learn how to focus their emotional energy. But what they are most excited about is their decision to use humor to manage the emotional swings. They have agreed to start singing when things are getting too emotional and also to take dancing lessons to focus this energy.

They make sure to establish a plan that they both feel is manageable and a method of measuring their progress. Just by deciding to work together and by putting the problem into simple language, Tamara and Kevin begin to feel more hopeful.

Kevin and Tamara came up with very good brainstorming solutions. Can you think of five more?

Meaningful activity focuses anxiety into a plan of action that mobilizes not only the patient but everyone around her. As the man, is it important that you create an environment where she can feel emotionally supported, deeply understood, and connected to you. But always remember that when it comes to menopause and cancer, you must be sure that the treating physician knows what is going on. There are effective medications to alleviate many of the symptoms associated with menopause.

We have covered a lot of information about menopause, but men tell us that this is a big challenge for them. No matter what happens, it is essential that you use COPE to help the woman and your family manage these unpleasant symptoms.

Non-Couple Relationships and Breast Cancer

This guide directs a lot of advice toward men who are in couple relationships with a woman with breast cancer. That doesn't mean that the many other men who care about her can't be just as helpful.

Helping Sisters, Mothers, and Other Women

A woman who has been diagnosed with breast cancer needs all the support she can get, particularly if she is not in a partner relationship. It can be difficult to know what is appropriate and what is intrusive, but the best way to find out is to offer to get involved. Don't be afraid to show that you care.

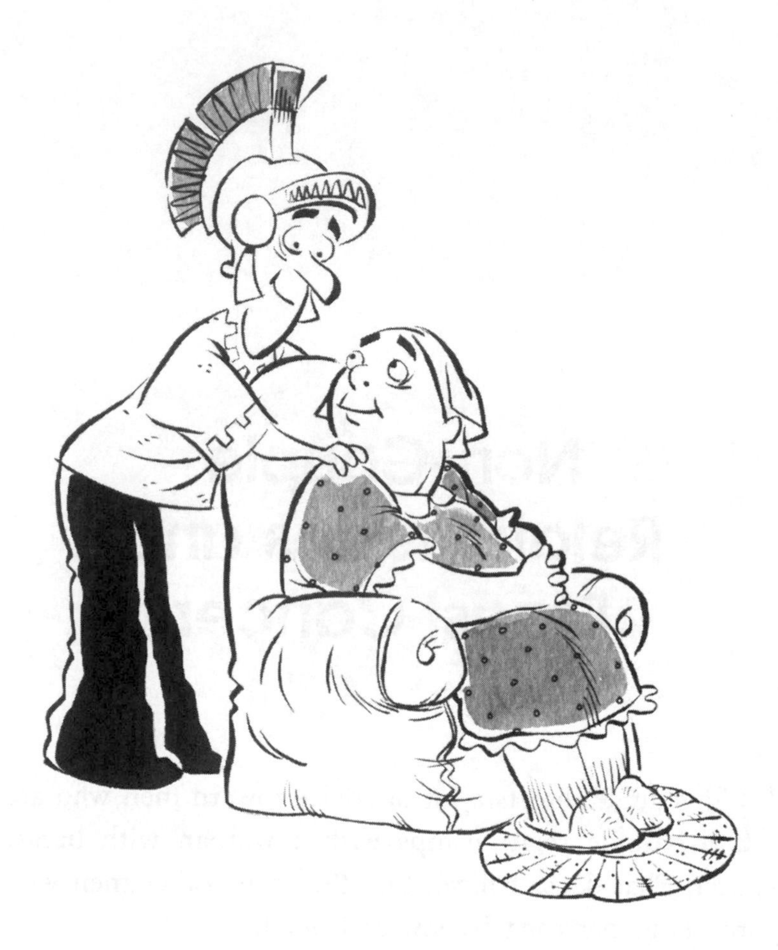

Advice for brothers, sons-in-law, and grandsons

Brothers, sons and grandsons often feel confused about how to best help the women in their lives when they are vulnerable. (This gets even harder if the woman with breast cancer is a stepmother or if there is a stepfather on the scene.) Although sons and grandsons often love their mothers and grandmothers very deeply, they sometimes feel distanced by the difference between how women and men choose to show concern and love. Generational differences can also make communication more difficult.

Not wanting to bother her is a pretty weak excuse for staying away during her time of need, so forget it! Let her tell you if she is too tired or not up to receiving your efforts. Even then, don't feel embarrassed or discouraged. Keep offering to help—she's sure to appreciate it.

Since men tend to avoid situations in which they feel they can't make a meaningful contribution, here are some suggestions on how to be helpful:

- Visit her whenever possible. Gifts are nice, but your presence will mean much more.
- Maintain telephone, e-mail, letter, or some other contact if you cannot be physically present.
- Call first—don't wait to be called.
- Talk with your father and siblings about how you can both work together to best support your mother.
- Be honest. Trying to protect women from the truth only makes them feel more alone.
- Tell her that you love her and that you would like to be helpful to her.
- Ask her about the breast cancer experience, and make sure she knows she can tell you anything, good or bad.
- Offer to accompany her to medical visits.
- Invite your mother to lunch, dinner, or some other social event.
- If you have children of your own, ask if she would like to spend time with them. If she says yes, be sure to follow through.

Advice for fathers, grandfathers, uncles, and other committed men

It can be really hard to know what to do for the woman you love who has breast cancer when you are not the husband or a son. Because other men are often not as close to the woman, it can be difficult for fathers, grandfathers, uncles, other relatives, and friends to know what kind of help will be welcome and what might be seen as pushy or invasive of her privacy.

However, you have a very important role to play. You can be extremely important in supporting not only the woman with breast cancer, but also her husband and/or son. Men frequently lack confidantes, and the men closest to her might appreciate someone to talk to.

Do not wait to be asked for help. Telling yourself that she or her immediate family will call you if they need you is a cop-out. Offer first, and let them tell you if they do or don't need your assistance.

Avoid rehashing any conflict that may have soured or limited your communication in the past, unless you feel you need to clear the air before you can be supportive. Even in that case, don't bring it up unless she seems willing. It might be too stressful for her, so try to gauge her reaction.

Once you've made contact, let her know that you are concerned and thinking of her. Offer to have lunch or dinner with her, or with her primary caregiver(s). If you have the resources, she and her family would probably greatly appreciate any kind of commitment: time, money, an apartment close to the hospital, medical and legal expertise, or transportation to and from treatments.

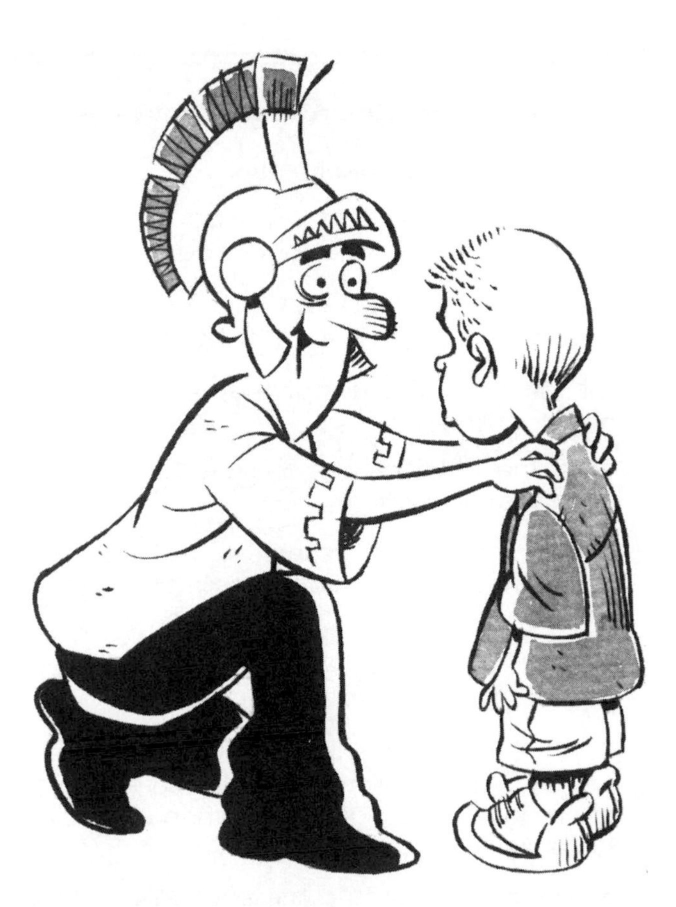

Children and Breast Cancer

Because most men instinctively protect (and overprotect) the people they love, children are all too often kept in the background when a family member is ill. This is almost always a bad idea. Depending on the age and maturity of the child, it is essential to provide him or her with realistic and accurate information that is age appropriate.

Providing age appropriate information means only asking the child to do things that make sense given the emo-

Talking to Children About Breast Cancer

Helpful techniques

- Share information that will impact the child using age-appropriate language
- Reassure the child that you will always be available to explain what is happening
- Tell the child that when people get sick, it's no one's fault
- Give the child plenty of time to understand complex information
- Encourage open expression of feelings. Say that it is normal and healthy to talk about sadness and to cry
- Always offer but never pressure the young person to talk
- Buy books that explain to children why people get sick and may die (make sure they are of an age-appropriate level), then discuss them together
- Be quick to speak to a mental health counselor when you are in doubt

Unhelpful techniques

- Tell the boy that he is now the man of the house
- Tell the girl that she is now the woman of the house
- Suggest that if the child behaves, the sick woman is likely to get well sooner
- Imply that the child caused the illness in any way
- Tell a child that a person who has died is sleeping

tional and intellectual maturity of a person of that age. For example, a child of three only understands situations as they pertain to his or her immediate situation, safety and needs, and that's normal. Very simple language and very small amounts of information over a period of day, weeks, or months is best. Gently ask if the child has any questions. Over time, a child who feels safe will ask questions. It is also helpful to ask the child what they understand about the situation so you can correct any misinformation. Always be honest—children can sense when you aren't telling the truth. And always, always be extremely patient. If you don't know what to say, a mental health professional will be able to guide you.

It is important to ask a child what he or she understands about the situation, then to fill in the gaps to demonstrate that you will be honest. At times, it is helpful to let the older child (eight years or older) or adolescent meet with the doctor, nurse, or social worker. Communication is essential to young people of all ages. Even if they're old enough to know better, they need to be reminded that they will not get sick, and that someone will always be there for them.

Children are experts at sensing the emotional climate in the family, and they know when something is wrong. Don't try to hide it. If *you* don't provide emotional support and the necessary information, the child will fill in the blanks with misperceptions gleaned from television, friends, or his or her imagination. Psychologically speaking, this can be very dangerous. Children tend to believe the world revolves around them, so they are quite likely to think (or at least wonder if) they caused the stress and sadness their family is suffering. Some children carry the mistaken belief that they have caused the illness or death of a loved one into adulthood. Also, an unexplained loss in early life can lead to feelings of guilt, shame, and to the inability to form close emotional attachments many years later. Unless thoughtful, loving adults step in, a child's emotional scars could last a lifetime. This is serious business.

Keeping the Romance In Your Relationship

In one of Men Against Breast Cancer's many national workshops, called "Partners in Survival," one of the participants expressed frustration about the trouble he had talking about sex with his wife, who was completing a round of chemotherapy. Across the room, a large, burly man spoke up.

"You make love to a woman over an entire lifetime," he said warmly. The other men nodded in agreement.

Later, we invited the women to join. (The men are told at the beginning of the workshops that if every single man agrees, the women can join us for the final thirty minutes. If anybody would rather not, we don't do it, no questions asked.)

A twenty-six-year-old mother told the men how her husband had supported her. Every day he had told her how

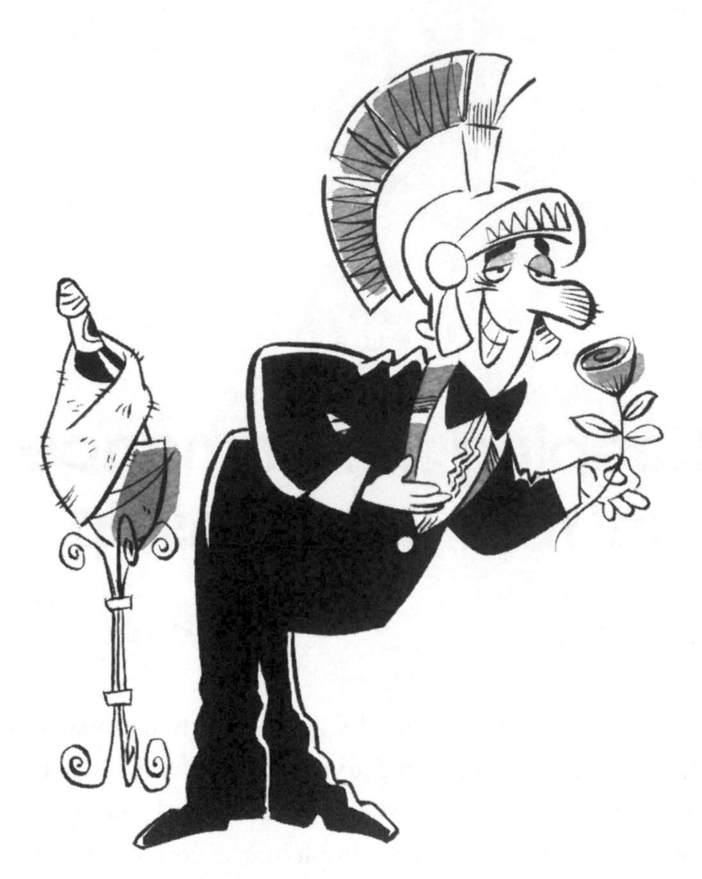

much he loved her and how beautiful she was. She said she knew her appearance had changed dramatically, but that her husband's love made her feel protected and respected.

One of the most important benefits of her husband's support, she added, was how comfortable she felt showing him her mastectomy scar. She didn't have to worry about upsetting him because she knew he would act like the strong man he truly was.

You make love to a woman over an entire lifetime. You're damn right, you do!

Women think about sex as much as men do, but they tend to think of it within a larger context of intimacy. In almost all cases, it is the man who has trouble bringing up changes and problems in a couple's sex life. Generally, women are very willing to talk about sex, but may also keep fears and feelings of guilt secret to avoid friction and shelter the man from embarrassment.

But keeping secrets about personal needs and concerns is always a bad idea. It takes too much energy to maintain a lie, and ignoring the situation won't make it go away and won't protect the other person. In fact, the person who claims to be "protecting" the other is usually just afraid to face facts.

The truth is that when (not *if*) the truth comes out, past secrecy will probably make the problem more hurtful and harder to resolve. All your energy, and hers, should be focused on mutual support, and that can only happen in the setting of honest and open communication.

Even if you think your situation is hopeless—she's in too much pain or is too tired to make love, you feel too depressed to maintain an erection, et cetera—there are still lots of ways to have a meaningful relationship, even sexually. This is the time to maximize your potential satisfaction by focusing on the bigger picture of intimacy, rather than struggling to continue the same sexual habits you've always had. This is the time to appreciate each other's bodies in a whole new way.

Getting Intimate

Sexual intimacy is the purest form of communication. In addition to intercourse, it may include hugging, kissing, spooning, touching, and sleeping side by side. Non-physical intimacy, such as writing love notes and reliving shared intimate experiences, can also be very stimulating.

Every couple has a unique sex life. The frequency and type of intimacy you engage in with a spouse or lover will probably fluctuate over time, but chances are good that sex will always be an important part of your life. Most people place high value on sexual identity in relationships, and breast cancer shouldn't force you and the woman you love to give that up.

Because speaking frankly about sex in public settings is not usually socially acceptable, exaggerated media portrayals have become our most visible models of intimacy. But although you've probably figured out by now that sex in the real world has its ups, downs, and limitations, a crisis in your sex life can make it easy to lose perspective. This section can help you understand what kinds of changes to expect and how to deal with them.

When Intimacy Just Isn't Happening

It is simply not possible to separate physical and emotional concerns when it comes to sexuality. Cancer and its treatments cause physical changes that can inhibit sexual desire and function, while stress and fear (emotional concerns) can easily hinder the body's ability to function properly, in both women (mostly decreased desire or lack of lubrication) and men (decreased desire or lack of an erection). Therefore, the origin of any problem you are experiencing may not be clear-cut.

Some men avoid sexual intimacy because they are afraid of hurting the woman. Women with breast cancer sometimes feel too embarrassed by their appearance to be intimate. There are any number of reasons why a couple in your situation might find their love life coming to a halt. It is important to remember that such struggles are normal and that there is *always* something you can do to improve matters, beginning with—you guessed it—communication.

Talking About Intimacy

Most women are more comfortable talking about sex than men, especially when it comes to analyzing problems and complexities. They tend to have a larger network of family and friends with whom they can communicate about intimate subjects, in very detailed terms. Many men only talk about sex with their partner, and those conversations are often too stifled to be helpful.

You don't need to discuss your sex life with outsiders, but you will need to expose your vulnerabilities and swallow your pride. You should know that even health care professionals can be reluctant to talk about sex, so it's up to you to get the conversation going.

That's right—not only are you going to have to talk about intimacy, but *you* have to be the one to bring it up. Waiting for a woman with breast cancer to bring up such a difficult topic is a cop-out. She's embarrassed, scared, and insecure right now, and silence will intensify those feelings. Help her out.

Questions to ask her

- What has changed for her due to cancer? Has her level of desire or comfort zone changed? What about physical changes?
- Would it be acceptable for her to show you those physical changes, like a surgical scar? Encourage her to do so. Once she shows you, there will be no surprises left. If there is a scar, it's best to be present at the first dressing.
- Is she still comfortable with having sex? What about other sexual activity, kissing, or hugging? Her objections, if she has any, might have either physical or emotional causes.
- Are you providing her with what she needs? Try not to get defensive if she says no. Complete honesty is best for your relationship.
- Is there anything she would like to tell or ask you? She might need prompting.

Women usually gravitate toward those who make them feel heard and understood. With a little effort and willingness, that can be you. Ultimately, open communication should lessen the tension between you and help you resume a more normal sex life. In most circumstances, a straightforward exchange of information about your feelings and apprehensions will make a big difference. But if you encounter a problem that you find too difficult to resolve, reach out for professional help.

Common Cancer-Related Sexual Problems

Impotence

Okay, so this is a sensitive issue for most guys. But as you probably know, impotence is not uncommon, especially in stressful situations. You shouldn't be surprised if achieving an erection is more difficult than usual.

- Have sex earlier in the day
- Begin with oral sex
- Use medications—hey, it worked for Bob Dole!
- Take a warm shower or bath
- Get more exercise
- Avoid alcohol and cigarettes
- Talk to a physician, nurse, or social worker

Vaginal Drying

Just as you might have some trouble getting going, the woman might also need some assistance. Don't think it means she isn't interested in sex. Some of the same tactics that work for you might help her, too. Try these ideas:

- Have sex earlier in the day
- Begin with oral sex
- Only have oral sex
- Use lubricants or moisturizers (for example, Astrogilde or VagiFem), but avoid products that are not specifically manufactured for sexual activity such as petroleum jelly, which can cause infection
- Use medications for vaginal lubrication
- Massage her gently in a circular motion with your fingers

- Take a warm shower or bath together
- Talk with a physician about local estrogen (cream or E-string)

A Recipe for Romance

Nothing sparks romance like a well-prepared, savory meal. No one knows this better than Jacques Haeringer, the chef de cuisine of the nationally-known restaurant L'Auberge Chez François in Great Falls, Virginia. Chef Jacques always insists on using the purest of ingredients, both for taste and health.

Jacques first joined the battle against breast cancer when his wife, Evelyn, was diagnosed with the disease. He suggests this recipe from his book *Two for Tonight.** Personally prepared by you, it's sure to help rekindle your love life.

Beef Rib Baked in a Salt Crust and Gratin of Spinach and Mushrooms

Since prehistoric times, salt has been a precious commodity—probably one of the oldest commodities traded by man. The Hebrews used it in sacrifices and ceremonies. Homer described nations as poor when they did not have salt to season their food. The Romans used salt to preserve fish, olives, cheese, and meat and it formed part of the soldiers' wages. In this recipe, I use sea salt (the most nutritious and pure) to form a crust that seals in the juices of the beef and yields an amazing tenderness. I recommend

*Jacques E. Haeringer, *Two for Tonight: Pure Romance from L'Auberege François.* (Silver Spring, MD: Bartleby Press, 2001), 180.

sea salt of unrefined mineral salt. Both contain all the vital trace minerals which are often processed out of ordinary table salt.

The Gratin of Spinach and Mushrooms:

½ pound spinach
4 ounces white mushrooms
2 tablespoons butter
1 teaspoon finely minced shallots
⅔ cup heavy whipping cream
1 egg yolk
¼ teaspoon of freshly ground nutmeg
Sea Salt or unrefined
Freshly ground pepper

The Beef:

1 16-18 ounce boneless rib-eye
1 teaspoon cracked peppercorns
1 pound coarse sea or kosher salt
4 ounces all-purpose flour
¾ cup water

To Prepare the Gratin

- Wash several times, de-stem, and thoroughly drain (pat dry) the spinach leaves.
- Wash the mushrooms by placing in a large bowl of water. Lift the mushrooms out of the bowl leaving the grit behind.
- *Preheat oven to 400 degrees*
- Melt 1 tablespoon of butter in a small sauté pan, when the butter beings to foam, add ½ of the

shallots; stir into the butter and add the spinach leaves. Cook for approximately 1 minute to just wilt the spinach. Set aside.

- Slice the mushrooms.
- Wipe the sauté pan clean; melt the remaining table spoon of butter. When the butter begins to foam, add the remaining shallots; stir into the butter and slice mushrooms. Sauté for 1-2 minutes until just cooked through.
- With the aid of a rubber spatula, transfer the mushrooms to a small oven-proof dish. Place the cooked spinach over the mushrooms.
- Place the egg yolk in a small mixing bowl and whisk thoroughly. Add the cream, nutmeg, salt, and pepper blending completely.
- Pour the egg/cream combination over the vegetables. Place the dish in a preheated 400-degree oven for 5-7 minutes until nicely browned.

To Prepare the Beef

- *Preheat the oven to 500 degrees*
- Trim any excess fat and silver skin from the beef.
- Season the beef with the cracked peppercorns.
- Mix the salt and flour together in a bowl and add the water to obtain a moderately thick paste.
- Using the heel of your hand, firmly press the paste around the beef, forming a salt crust.
- Place the beef on a backing sheet and place in the preheated oven for approximately 10 minutes. Reduce heat to 450 degrees and bake another 10 min-

utes for medium-rare. Remove the beef from the oven and allow to rest for 10-12 minutes.

To Serve

- Present in the beef and break away from the crust with the aid of a large kitchen spoon or spatula.
- Place on a cutting board and slice diagonally.
- Serve at once with the Gratin of Spinach and Mushrooms and a Madeira Sauce if desired.

Applying the COPE Model

The COPE Model will help you talk about resuming or enhancing romantic activities, sexual and otherwise. The sexual problems you choose to address might be biological, psychological, interpersonal, or any combination thereof.

Creativity

Just being open to new ideas about sex can be a big help. Lots of couples come to a comfortable place in their sex life and stop thinking of it as dynamic and evolving. Don't be afraid to suggest new ideas, and make sure you ask the woman if she has any ideas of her own. With creativity comes an atmosphere of fun and experimentation that can really lighten the mood. Stress is a sex-killer!

Now that you have a brainstorming system, you might even find yourself automatically thinking of creative solutions to your problems. If so, great! Give yourself enough rein to explore all the possibilities.

Optimism

A sex-related problem can be discouraging, but if you

and the woman have been together for any length of time, you probably have some experience and know that any partnership is going to have ups and downs.

Focus on your goal. There is no room for negativity or fear. Remember that, generally speaking, even the most successful people have plenty of failures. But you only become a failure yourself when you give up trying.

Planning

Like explaining a good joke, thinking too much about sex can kill the mood. But in this case, a little forethought (before the foreplay) is advised. How far do you want to go? Are you both mentally prepared to face changes and difficulties you've never experienced before? What are you going to do or say if something isn't working?

Expert Information

As always, the health care team is an excellent source of information about physical effects of cancer that might influence the woman's sex life. But ultimately, the woman herself provides the expert information. For help adapting to the changes in your relationship, try a counselor.

Maybe you find it strange or uncomfortable to have to work harder at something that once have came more easily. But although cancer complicates romance and sex, there is a silver lining: feeling more intimate with the woman you love than you ever imagined possible. Being forced to talk more openly and honestly might seem awkward at first, but over time you will be amazed at how good you will feel when you are deeply connected to the most important person in your life.

Survivorship: Life After Breast Cancer

Who Is a Cancer Survivor?

Each year 1.2 million Americans are diagnosed with cancer. Over ten million men and women are living with cancer in the United States today. But these numbers don't include everyone who has had to manage the stress of real and potential losses associated with cancer, or the psychological and financial uncertainty that come from treatment. They don't include family members and other loved ones. They don't include *you.*

This is an important point to make, because when a loved one is ill, we men tend to minimize our own emotional distress. As a man, you can play a very powerful role in supporting the woman in your life's efforts to manage her concerns and fears.

Opportunities for Men

What man wouldn't feel sad, angry, frustrated, and confused when a woman he loves is sick and at risk of dying? Sometimes we have to ignore our own distress to make the people in our lives feel safe and secure, but sometimes doing this just makes them feel alone. It teaches our sons and daughters a dishonest and unhealthy way of coping with life's problems. Courage is being able to demonstrate commitment while being open and honest about concerns for the future.

The time after the woman has completed treatment is difficult for everyone and can be very confusing. You might feel safer if you maintain a connection with health care providers. After a long and intense period of medical care, not seeing a doctor can be scary. Here are a few reasons why:

- Because we always feel a need to do something, once treatment ends our sense of direction is lost.
- Although worry generally decreases over time, the fear of recurrence is always high when treament stops because the patient is no longer under extremely careful monitoring.
- The supportive relationship with the health care team (physician, nurse, social worker, staff and others) is lessened. For someone who might never have experienced such a caring relationship, this can be a big emotional loss.
- As the focus on treatment and monitoring fades, the realties of life resurface in full force.
- When active treatment stops, people have time to

assess how much it has cost them and their families. The price is always high, and so might be the guilt.

As the demands of cancer treatment fade, the woman may begin to think about how her cancer has affected her life, both outwardly and inwardly. She might question family relationships and her occupational choice. It is normal to be nervous about what could happen as a result of this reassessment, but she needs you to see things from her perspective.

The uncertainty of cancer is difficult for everyone. Since treatments can last months or even years, patients and their loved ones might have assumed new roles in the family structure. These changes are hard even if they have good consequences. For example, if an adolescent daughter has taken on some of her mothers responsibilities, she may not want to give them up when her mother is ready to resume her role. This can make the mother feel replaced and/or unneeded, and can also make the daughter feel rejected.

Those affected by cancer will carry reminders of it for the rest of their lives. The long-term effects of treatments can include permanent physical changes such as menopausal symptoms, cognitive dysfunction, fatigue, and sexual problems. Fear, anxiety, and depression are also common. If woman has children she will often worry about their health. Because the genetics of cancer are complex, there is a lot of confusion about what predisposition actually means for the family. However, having one blood relative with cancer means a child is more likely to develop cancer. Knowing this is a hard and might make the survivor feel guilty. Ask your physician to explain the benefits of genetic counseling in your particular situation.

Maximizing Normalcy: Honesty and Connection

Life is never the same after cancer, but affected people will find that once the immediate threat of the disease is over and "normal" life comes back into focus, the important things—family, work, and friends—re-emerge.

You must remember that women find it helpful to talk about their concerns. That doesn't mean they expect you to fix all the issues they raise. They don't want to be controlled by you; rather, they want to feel connected to you. Remember that women need to know that they are loved and respected. They seldom understand the shame men feel for being unable to protect loved ones from harm. Your inclination to ignore what cannot be controlled and avoid shame can leave the woman feeling alone and isolated. Be open and honest with each other—when you share, you'll feel much more deeply connected. The cancer experience can give you a new chance to learn about each other and feel united in ways you never imagined possible.

Returning to Work

Research shows that most cancer survivors are able to return to work and to make major contributions. However, there is a series of problems related to this return. It is almost always helpful to keep her boss informed of when the woman will be able to go back to work. Remember, her boss might not understand the reality of cancer survivorship. Share just enough information for her boss to know that the woman will still be a productive and reliable employee.

Your own colleagues might be uncomfortable talking to you about your situation. You can help put them at ease by preparing a short "go-to" statement, such as, "My wife [daughter, mother, sister] is off treatment now and is doing as well as can be expected."

You might want to share more information with people you feel close to, but remember that some people are scared of cancer. They might have had bad experiences with it that will make them act irrationally now. Try to remember how hard it is for people when they want to be helpful but are too burdened by their own fears to be effective.

At times it may seem like everyone has something to say about cancer. Be it a horror story, far-off cure, or opinion on how you should be handling your situation, it could make you feel like you are not doing enough. You might have to tell people, "I know you are trying to be helpful, but we are happy with our plan. When you keep telling me what we should do, it makes me unsure about what we're already doing and less confident in our health care team."

Again, finances are also a major concern for most people who are going back to work. Half of all bankruptcies in the United States are caused by medical debt, so it is essential to maintain health insurance. Today, fewer jobs are offering insurance, and those that do are asking employees to pay more out of pocket. If you have questions, talk with an expert early on. Some people will change their priorities once cancer treatment ends, but it is important not to change jobs until health coverage is made clear. Don't assume anything; people *do* lose health insurance. And once a person with cancer loses his or her health insurance, it is very hard to get it back.

Support and educational groups share ways to manage the demands of returning to work, especially how to adocate with insurance companies. The Wellness Community is one of the most popular free, nationally-run groups. You and the woman should go to at least one of these meetings so you can learn how others in your position have managed.

For more information, learn about Americans with Disabilities Act. It has a lot of helpful information about going back to work.

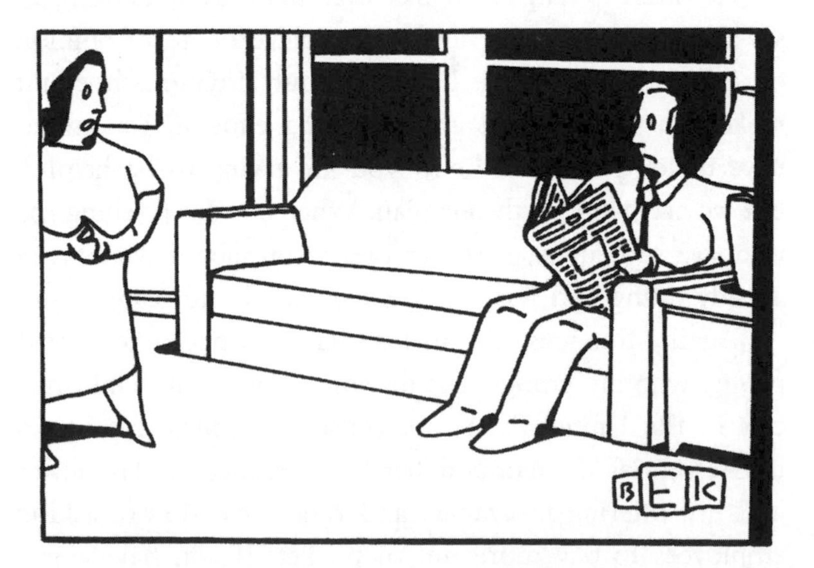

"Can you spare a few seconds to minimize my problems?"

Managing Physical Symptoms

Many women will experience physical changes and symptoms as a result of cancer or its treatment that will require ongoing attention. Varying levels of changes in thinking and memory ("chemo-brain"), fatigue, insomnia, hot flashes, swelling, weight changes, reduced sex drive, vaginal drying, anxiety, depression, and pain are common. Lymphedema (fluid retention, or swelling, as a result of surgery to the lymph channels in the arm) is also a common physical problem for which the woman and man are often ill-prepared.

You can play an important role in learning what to expect and where to find help. Men are superb advocates and really know how to hunt up relevant information. In all of these circumstances, it is important to seek out professional help—the sooner, the better! There are experts in all of these areas. Your physician, nurse, or social worker should be able to give you specific names and contact information. Men, don't allow anyone to minimize the woman's concerns. This is all too common, especially, unfortunately, with male physicians. Be sure to seek a second opinion if the woman's problems are not addressed. Survivorship is harder if suffering is not well-managed.

Ask for Help!

Men often find it difficult to ask for help, but it takes courage to accept your own fears and doubts while still moving forward. It also takes guts to accept your personal anxieties by parlaying them into meaningful activity. True wisdom is needed to engage a woman who is focused on her fear. But it takes no courage, none at all, to run away from responsibilities and deny emotions.

Don't ignore your emotional needs. Always be honest with yourself as well as the woman in your life. Connection to others is something we all desire, but it varies from person to person. If you feel sexually frustrated, miss playing golf, or are concerned about money, just say so—you can be sure she already knows. But not talking about it makes you seem too emotionally fragile to deal with. If you can't find the right words or are just too upset to tell her how you feel, talk to a counselor. It will probably only take one or two sessions, and it will help your relationship and you as an individual. If you need help finding a counselor in your area who specializes in cancer, go to the American Psychological Oncology Society website (see the Resources listed at the back of this book).

When You Have to Say Goodbye

Women are the center of family life. This is no exaggeration. They are often in charge of our social life and tend to be more interactive with our children than we do. So when a wife, sister, or daughter dies, the men who loved her grieve very deeply and are likely to become isolated. They often become depressed and are more at risk for illness than women who experience the death of a man. For men, what they see as their failure to protect the most important person in their life leads to an overwhelming sense of shame and grief.

It is important to be honest with your loved ones and yourself about the woman who is dying. This honesty creates a level of emotional and spiritual connection that gives the woman a sense of safety, even in the face of imminent separation and loss. Survivorship must now be measured not by how long she lives, but by the quality of her relationships and meaningfulness of her life. As a man, you can help to create a safe and loving environment in which courage supplants fear and sadness becomes a catalyst for deeper nuturing and healing.

For men who are able to control their fear and overwhelming feelings, this is an opportunity for emotional growth. You can reflect on your relationship and grieve for the loss of the woman and your dreams of a future life together. You will also have a much greater likelihood of having a healthy future relationship with another woman. But if you ignore your emotions and/or quickly replace the woman to avoid your feelings, your loss will *not* become an opportunity for growth and wisdom.

Children are often deeply disturbed and bewildered when their father (in their view) tries to replace their mother. This can create a lack of trust and a lot of confusion that isolate the man even more. Avoidance, addiction, depression, and anger might all be expressions of underlying grief.

Generally speaking, unless plans have already been made beforehand, you should not make any major changes in your life for a year after the death of a loved one. The period after the death of a loved one should be seen as an altered state of consciousness—one in which bad decisions are too often made.

The COPE Model, as described throughout this book,

can help you manage the period after the woman's death. Although no one can take away the pain and sorrow you will feel, meaningful activities (especially with immediate family and friends) can help to heal some of the suffering and ensure wiser decisions. Engaging your family or friends in using the COPE Model to best manage problems together will deepen family connections and allow you to teach your children how to effectively cope with one of life's most difficult and forseeable problems.

If you do not have any close family members or friends, attend a support group for men who have experienced the death of a loved one. You can see a professional counselor, too. You might be surprised to find out how many resources are available to you. Just call the nearest non-profit hospice or the department of social work. Use these resources before your loved one dies or as close to her death as possible.

Some day we will all die. The death of a cherished loved one may be the most difficult time we will ever face. This is one challenge you do not want to minimize, avoid, or deny. How you cope with loss is in your control, and by grieving honestly so that you can go on living a meaningful life, you will set a much-needed example for family, friends, and others. That is truly a courageous act.

Applying the COPE Model

Not knowing what the future brings makes most of us nervous. Cancer takes away our sense of safety and security and makes us realize just how limited life really is. It is important that families have an ongoing commitment to one another, no matter what happens. Research shows that a woman with breast cancer copes better with the support of her partner and family. So your input has a direct effect on how she manages her concerns and fears about cancer.

Courageous men in doubt use the COPE Model to solve their problems. If the problem is helping the woman in our life cope with the fear of recurrence, we can use COPE to manage it.

The Problem

How can you help the woman with breast cancer cope with the uncertainty of her situation?

Expert information

What specifically does the woman say about her fears? What type of fear is it—is she afraid of recurrence, death, money, returning to work, the health of her family? What techniques does she already use to manage her fears?

Creativity

Without passing judgment, create a list of ways to help the woman cope with her fears of uncertainty. This list will become an essential part of the planning process.

- Talk about it
- Hug each other
- Exercise
- Find distractions, i.e. movies, books, museums
- Limit your exposure to the mass media

- Surround yourself with supportive people
- Schedule times when you can talk about your feelings and concerns
- Explore new hobbies
- Learn to find meaning in your lives (read books, have conversations, take courses, etc.)
- Join advocacy groups to improve health care for yourself and others
- Learn relaxation and meditation techniques
- Write a book about your experience
- Keep a diary of your fears and grossly exaggerate them as much as possible, then each week burn them or flush them down the toilet
- Talk to your loved ones to find out how they would manage if your worst fears were realized
- Focus on living in the moment

Optimism

As always when using the COPE Model, it is essential to be optimistic as you persevere. Maintaining a positive outlook will help the woman and you replace your fear with hope.

Planning

It's time to look at the list and cross out any options you know your partner and you will not use. Always be honest with yourself; if you aren't, you will only be making things worse.

Choose options that will (1) give you the greatest potential benefit, (2) have the least amount of negative consequences or risk, and (3) take the least amount of effort. It is also helpful to think about what options you can and will act on over the following three to five days. You will find that just going through this exercise will decrease your fears and create a sense of control. More importantly, it will make the woman in your life feel deeply connected to you.

Conclusion

Relationships between men and women have always tested the boundaries of human connection. These relationships are challenging, volatile, and highly rewarding. In all cultures, the combination of the masculine and the feminine creates something that is greater than the sum of its parts, and not just in the literal sense. Beyond the miracle of creation, deep emotional and spiritual bonds can exist between mothers and sons, fathers and daughters, brothers and sisters, friends, and others. The intensity of these relationships springs directly from our genetic material—our gender synergy—as well as our commitment to each other.

We live in a time when the opportunities for women are increasing and the ways men define themselves are expanding. Wise and courageous people can turn their fear of change into excitement, rejecting schoolyard assumptions about what it means to be a man or a woman. There are no limits to the options they give themselves and each other. You can make the decision to base your own relationships on mutual regard, unconditional love, and respect for the diversity of human perspectives and behaviors that ultimately strengthens us all.

By taking the time to read *For the Women We Love*, you have already decided what kind of man you will be. It takes curiosity and courage to be open to new ideas. Learning to use the COPE model and finding out how to get the best out of your masculinity are acts with major implications for the next generation as they, too, learn how to work together as a team within an evolving context of profound respect and collaboration. You can honestly say that you are helping create a new concept of "manhood" to which we should all aspire as we learn how to support and care for the women we love.

Cancer has a way of focusing the mind and clearing away the noise. Those who are willing to listen will hear the harmony of men and women working together.

C.O.P.E. Practice Session Worksheet

Define Problem in simple words

____

____

- Something you really care about
- Your life will get better if you manage this better
- Can be influenced by you

Expert Information

What you need to know about this problem to better understand how to solve or manage the problem

______________________ ______________________
______________________ ______________________
______________________ ______________________
______________________ ______________________
______________________ ______________________

Creativity (brainstorm – generating as many creative ways to solve this problem <u>without judging any options</u>)

Optimism (focusing on the positive; expect to succeed)

Planning (From the list of brainstorming options, eliminate options with negative consequences, include options that are likely to succeed, choose the easiest.)

Resources

American Cancer Society
800.227.2345
www.cancer.org
P.O. Box 22718
Oklahoma City, OK 73123-1718

Breastcancer.org
www.breastcancer.org
breastcancer.org
111 Forrest Avenue 1R
Narberth, PA 19072

Cancer Care, Inc.
800.813.4673
www.cancercare.org
275 Seventh Avenue
New York, NY 10001

Cancer and Careers: Living and Working with Cancer
www.cancerandcareers.org

Community Breast Health Project
650.326.6686
www.med.stanford.edu
390 Cambridge Avenue
Palo Alto, CA 94306

Dr. Susan Love's Website for Women
www.susanlovemd.org
1.310.230.1712 Ext. 23
Dr. Susan Love Research Foundation
875 Via De La Paz, Ste. C
Pacific Palisades, CA 90272.

Family Caregiver Alliance
1.800.445.8106
www.caregiver.org
180 Montgomery Ste. 1100
San Francisco, CA 94104

Gilda's Club
(888) GILDA-4-U
www.gildasclub.org
322 Eighth Avenue, Ste. 1402
New York, NY 10001

Hospice Foundation of America
1.800.854.3402
www.hospicefoundation.org
12000 Biscayne Boulevard #505
Miami, FL 33181

Kids Konnected
1.800.899.2866
www.kidskonnected.org
27071 Cabot Road Ste. 102
Laguna Hills, CA 92653

Lance Armstrong Foundation
1.866.235.7205
www.livestrong.org
PO Box 161150
Austin, TX 78716-1150

Living Beyond Breast Cancer
1.888.753.5222
www.lbbc.org
10 East Athens Avenue, Ste. 204
Ardmore, PA 19003

Look Good Feel Better
1.800.395-LOOK
www.lookgoodfeelbetter.org
1101 17th Street Ste. 300
Washington, DC 20036

Men Against Breast Cancer
1.866.547.6222
www.menagainstbreastcancer.org
PO Box 150
Adamstown, MD 21710-0150

Mothers Supporting Daughters with Breast Cancer
410.778.1982
www.mothersdaughters.org
25235 Foxchase Drive
Chestertown, MD 21620-3409

National Breast Cancer Coalition
1.800.622.2838
www.natlbcc.org
1101 17th Street, NW, Ste. 1300
Washington, DC 20036

National Alliance of Breast Cancer Organizations
1.888.806.2226
www.nabco.org

National Alliance for Hispanic Health
202.387.5000
www.hispanichealth.org
1501 16th Street, NW
Washington, DC 20036

National Asian Women's Health Organization
415.989.9747
www.nawho.org

National Black Leadership Initiative on Cancer
1.800.724.1185
www.nblic.org
720 Westview Drive, SW
Atlanta, GA 30310

National Comprehensive Cancer Network
1.888.909.6226
www.nccn.org
500 Old York Road, Ste. 250
Jenkintown, PA 19046

National Coalition for Cancer Survivorship
1.877.622.7937
www.canceradvocacy.org

National Family Caregivers Association
1.800.896.3650
www.thefamilycaregiver.org
10400 Connecticut Avenue, Ste. 500
Kensington, MD 20895-3944

National Hospice and Palliative Care Organization
1.800.658.8898
www.nhpco.org
1700 Diagonal Road, Ste. 625
Alexandria, VA 22314

National Institutes of Health
301.496.4000
www.nih.gov
9000 Rockville Pike
Bethesda, MD 20892

Patient Advocate Foundation
1.800.532.5274
www.patientadvocate.org
700 Thimble Shoals Blvd, Ste. 200
Newport News, VA 23606

Partnership for Prescription Assistance
1.888.477.2669
www.pparx.org

People Living With Cancer
(Patient website of the American Society of Clinical Oncology)

www.plwc.org
1900 Duke Street, Ste. 200
Alexandria, VA 22314

SHARE
(Self-Help for women with breast or ovarian Cancer)
1.866.891.2392
www.sharecancersupport.org
1501 Broadway, Ste. 704A
New York, NY 10036

Sisters Network Inc.
1.866.781.1808
www.sistersnetworkinc.org
8787 Woodway Drive, Ste. 4206
Houston, TX 77063

Susan G. Komen Breast Cancer Foundation
1.800.462.9273
www.komen.org
Headquarters
5005 LBJ Freeway, Ste. 250
Dallas, TX 75244

The National Cancer Institute: Cancer Information Services
1.800.4.CANCER
www.cancer.gov

The Witness Project
1.800.275.1183
www.acrc.uams.edu/patients/witness_project

Ulman Cancer Fund for Young Adults
1.888.393-FUND
www.ulmanfund.org
PMB #505
4725 Dorsey Hall Drive, Ste. A
Ellicott City, MD 21042

Well Spouse Association
1.800.838.0879
www.wellspouse.org
63 West Main Street, Ste. H
Freehold, NJ 07728

Y-ME National Breast Cancer Organization
1.800.221.2141
www.y-me.org
212 W. Van Buren, Ste. 1000
Chicago, IL 60607-3903

Young Survival Coalition
212.206.6610
877-YSC-1011 (toll-free)
www.youngsurvival.org
61 Broadway, Ste. 2235
New York, NY 10006

You may also find the following publications useful:

Balch D. (2003) *Cancer for Two: An inspiring true story and guide for cancer patients and their partners..* A Few Good People, Inc.

Brown T. (2005) *Men Bleed Too. A compelling story about one man's struggle to help his wife fight breast cancer.* iUniverse press.

Garbowski, AJ, Shaw LJ. (2007) *Don't Walk Through the Mirror.* McMillen Publishing.

Golant M, Golant SK (2007) *What To Do When Someone You Love Is Depressed.* New York: Henry Holt and Company.

Hewitt M, Herdman R, Holland J. (Eds.) *Meeting Psychosocial Needs of Women with Breast Cancer.* Washington D.C.: The National Academies Press, 2004. (www.nap.edu)

Houts, PS. (Ed.) *Home Care Guide for Cancer.* American College of Surgeons, 1994.

Kneece JC. *Helping Your Mate Face Breast Cancer*: Tips for Becoming an Effective Support Partner. (4th Edition). Columbia, S.C.: EduCare Publishing, 2001 (www.cancerhelp.com)

Landay, D. (1998) *Be Prepared: The Complete Financial, Legal, and Practical Guide to Living with Cancer, HIV, and Life-Challenging Conditions.* New York: St Martin's Press.

Love P, Stosny S. (2007) *How to improve your marriage without talking about it: finding love beyond words.* New York: Broadway Books.

Martin TL, Doka KJ. (2000) *Men Don't Cry…Women Do.* Bruner/Mazel.

Nezu AM, Nezu CM, Friedman, SH, Faddis S. Houts PS. (1998)) *Helping Cancer Patients Cope.* American Psychological Association.

Silver M. (2004) *Breast Cancer Husband: How to Help Your Wife (and Yourself) Through Diagnosis, Treatment, and Beyond.* Rodale.

About Men Against Breast Cancer

Men Against Breast Cancer, co-founded by Marc Heyison and Stephen Peck in 1999, is the first national non-profit organization dedicated to educating and empowering men to be effective caregivers when breast cancer strikes a female loved one.

MABC recognizes that breast cancer not only has devastating effects on the affected woman but on her family as well, as demonstrated by our pink and blue ribbon symbolizing a partnership between men and women. Therefore, MABC's philosophy is to help the family help support the patient, with special emphasis on the important role of the primary male caregiver: the husband, brother, or father. At the same time, MABC deeply respects and recognizes that the ultimate decisions regarding treatment and care must be made by the patient.

With this in mind MABC's signature program, *Partners In Survival,* combines a blueprint to help navigate the crisis of breast cancer with a proven systematic approach to problem solving called the COPE Model, which is being taught all over the world.

The success of *Partners In Survival* was recognized when the Center's For Disease Control in 2003 awarded MABC the first ever grant to a men's organization to bring our innovative program to derserving communities throughout the country.

MABC is also letting the world know that men can and must play a critical role in being there for the women they love. We provide men with the opportunity to learn from each other as they redefine what it means to be a wise and courageous caregiver. By supporting the man, we are ultimately supporting the woman and improving her quality of life. And what could be more important than that?

For more information or to support MABC, please visit www.menagainstbreastcancer.org.

About the Authors

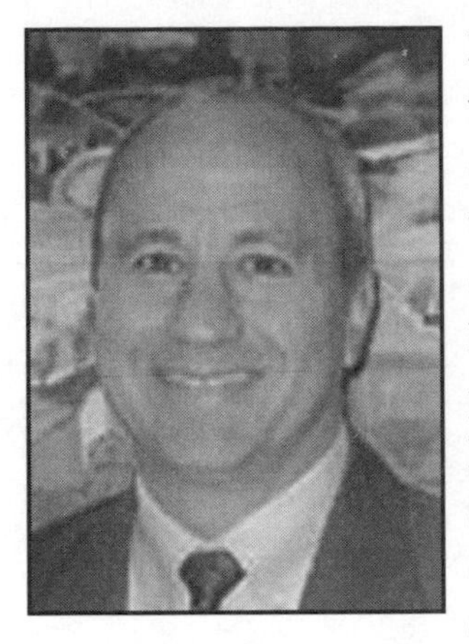

Matthew J. Loscalzo has over twenty-six years of professional expertise in strengths-based counseling of cancer patients and their families. His particular clinical and research interests focus on helping people to use systematic approaches to solve complex problems. He has also focused on developing Gender Synergies—ways that women and men can work together to get the best out of each other. Matthew has held leadership positions at Memorial Sloan-Kettering Cancer Center, The Johns Hopkins Oncology Center, and the Moores University of California at San Diego Cancer Center, and is now at the City of Hope as the Administrative Director of the Sheri and Les Biller Patient and Family Resource Center. He is an internationally recognized lecturer and has published many professional articles.

Marc Heyison is the president and co-founder of Men Against Breast Cancer. Since 1992, when his mother was diagnosed with breast cancer, his passion and mission in life has been to help others navigate the crisis of breast cancer. He is a nationally recognized speaker and expert in caregiving issues for men. Marc, a former professional baseball player, lives in Maryland with his wife Tanya and daughter Samantha.

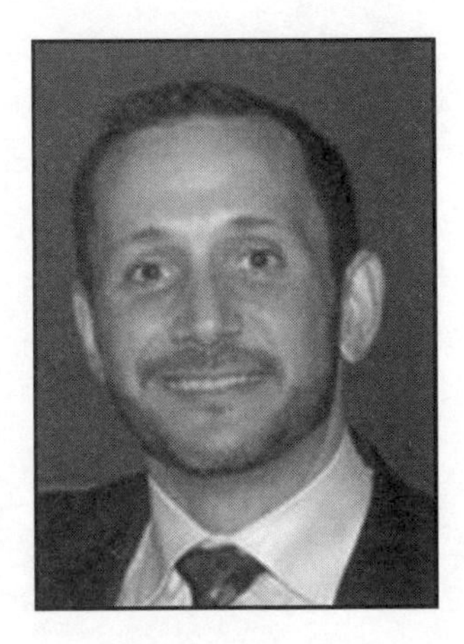

Important Information and Phone Numbers

Use this page to note phone numbers and other information that you will need over time. Some contacts might include physicians, nurses, social workers, and pharmacists.

Notes

Notes